kinesiology

"This is Stupid's Book"

GENE A. LOGAN

University of Southern California

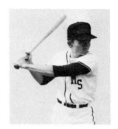

WAYNE C. McKINNEY

Southwest Missouri State College

kinesiology

Illustrated by Philip J. Van Voorst

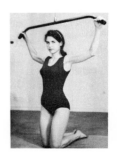

WM. C. BROWN COMPANY PUBLISHERS

PHYSICAL EDUCATION SERIES

Consulting Editor

AILEENE LOCKHART
University of Southern California
Los Angeles, California

Copyright © 1970 by
Wm. C. Brown Company Publishers

ISBN 0–697– 07107–3

Library of Congress Catalog Card Number: 74-106949

Third Printing, 1972

Printed in the United States of America

contents

APPENDIXES

preface

This basic kinesiology textbook is written for physical education majors. It is hoped that these future physical educators will use kinesiologic knowledge to help improve performances of their students. The motives for writing this book were to organize and to present existing kinesiologic subject matter in a more meaningful and effective manner, that is, to show the interrelationships between kinesiologic theory and practice. Many physical educators apparently consider kinesiology to be useful in theory only. In some colleges and universities, this subject has been treated too superficially or only as an academic exercise for the undergraduate student majoring in physical education. Such experiences are usually the beginning and end of kinesiology for the future educator. Kinesiology should be a daily "working tool" for the physical educator. Utilization of kinesiology is absolutely essential to properly teach activities found within professionally recognized programs and curricula in physical education departments.

Confusion often exists concerning the relationship of theory to practice. Arthur Schopenhauer, a nineteenth-century German philosopher, indicated that theoretical subject matter must have a sound, logical basis and must work in practice. If theory cannot be applied in practice, it is not good theory. Most kinesiologic theory has withstood the test of time. Consequently, physical educators should be able to use this knowledge as a basis for their teaching practices. When kinesiology theory is used in practice, the physical educator is more capable of helping the individual student attain his potential as a performer.

One of the major objectives of physical education is to develop the highest possible level of neuromuscular skill in individual students. This objective may be obtained most effectively by using kinesiologic techniques during the teaching-learning process. This book was designed and organized to assist the student in developing an understanding of the components of human motion. *There is a progression from basic kinesiologic subject matter to kinesiologic constructs to analyses of skills and, finally, to the improvement of performance.* The professional physical educator must have a functional knowledge of these facets of kinesiology if he is to be an effective teacher-coach.

Basic body movements and anatomic structures are discussed in Part One. Joint movements are presented and accompanied by illustrations of these movements. Selected anatomic landmarks and planes of movement are also presented. Since most kinesiology students have had a prerequisite course in human anatomy, no attempt has been made to duplicate and discuss all anatomic and bony landmarks within this book. Selected anatomic landmarks and bones are found in Appendix A.

The traditional planes of movement are shown. In addition, diagonal movement patterns, or the concept of *diagonal planes,* are introduced. The rationale underlying the need for diagonal planes is presented to facilitate communication regarding sports motion.

There is a detailed discussion of *applied myology* in Part Two. It is well established neurologically that muscles work in groups as opposed to working individually; consequently, the approach to myology in this book emphasizes muscle group or aggregate action. In addition, the concept of the interrelationship of several muscle groups working together in diagonal patterns to perform gross, sequential movement is introduced. This concept includes what is called the *serape effect* which is dependent, in part, upon a concept of muscle stabilization called *dynamic stabilization.* Owing to the aggregate action of muscles, joint movements are analyzed in terms of the *muscles most involved* in producing those motions. Terms such as "agonistic action," "prime movers," or "assistant movers" are not used.

The concept of the *spatial relationship of muscles to joints* is presented in detail. This approach to the study of muscle action allows the student to deduce logically the individual or aggregate muscle actions after the necessary anatomic concepts are known. This deemphasizes the importance of rote memory of muscle origins, insertions, and actions. Aggregate muscle actions are presented in Part Two, and individual—traditional—muscle attachments and actions are presented in Appendix B. The current *Nomina Anatomica* terminology is used in Appendix B.

Experience has indicated that students have considerable difficulty understanding the effect of gravity on muscle action when the body is in a variety of positions. As a result, there are several discussions (including examples), where appropriate throughout the text, of the effect of gravity on muscle actions in positions other than the classic anatomic position.

The authors have synthesized anatomic and mechanical principles into three large concepts called *kinesiologic constructs*: (1) summation of internal forces, (2) aerodynamics, and (3) hydrodynamics. These are presented in Part Three. A review of the kinesiologic literature reveals innumerable anatomic and mechanical facts related to human motion. This overwhelming number of facts combined with formulae from mathematics and physics tends to inhibit the learning of important kinesiologic constructs by physical education students. Therefore, the most pertinent of these facts have been synthesized into several workable kinesiologic constructs. This should serve as a *progression* into subsequent study of kinesiology and biomechanics.

Techniques for *noncinematographic and cinematographic analyses* as well as *segmental analysis techniques* are included. Comparative analyses of a skill are presented as examples of an important aspect of kinesiology introduced as *analytic kinesiology*. These are designed to serve as models for the physical educator who desires to know how to put kinesiologic theory into practice.

Improvement of performance is discussed by presenting basic elements of strength, flexibility, muscular endurance, and cardiovascular endurance development. These are the major factors underlying skill development. In addition, a new concept of improving performance, *Specifics,* is introduced.

Dr. Harold B. Falls, Jr., rates special consideration. It was he who suggested that we should write a kinesiology book designed to show the applicability of kinesiologic theory to practice in physical education.

Acknowledgment is made to the following individuals for their assistance as models for many of the illustrations: Bill Chapman, Bonus Frost, Tom Hodge, Ernie Jones, Jay Kinser, Bill Lamberson, Ardie McCoy, Mike McKinney, Ruth Miller, Andrea Morris, Sue Schuble, Alice Souther, and Jan Stevenson. Special acknowledgment is made to Sue Schuble for her contributions to the writing of Chapter 12. Finally, the work of Carol Garrison in preparing the manuscript is appreciated.

The content and purposes of the book, together with possible errors, are the sole responsibility of the authors.

Gene A. Logan
Wayne C. McKinney

study of human motion

Kinesiology is the study of human motion. The basic purposes of kinesiology are to provide the physical educator with (1) a professional understanding of human motion and (2) the ability to analyze human motion. The ability to analyze facilitates the teaching of neuromuscular skills and the selection of appropriate exercises and drills designed to improve performance. Thus, kinesiology provides the daily "working tools" for physical educators in their efforts to improve sport, exercise, and dance performances. This is one of the major objectives of physical education.

This basic text approaches kinesiology primarily from a functional point of view. There is an emphasis on the relationship between selected elements of myology and osteology as they relate to human motion. The most essential aspects of mechanics are synthesized into *kinesiologic constructs*. Furthermore, a special emphasis is placed on the practical application of kinesiologic theory in teaching-coaching situations. This is provided through discussions of noncinematographic and cinematographic analytic techniques, progressions for analyses, and selected models of analyses with implications and examples of specific exercises to improve performance.

Unlike many other kinesiology textbooks which contain separate discussions of such elements as gravity, equilibrium, motion, and force, there is an attempt to interweave these important elements in the text where they are functionally applicable. The attempt here is to make kinesiology "live" instead of providing a discussion of separate abstract entities which may or may not be applied in a meaningful manner to improve performance.

To be a professional physical educator—a man or woman who incorporates knowledge from the scientific, technical, and philosophic bases

1

of physical education in teaching and coaching situations—it is imperative that kinesiologic theory be applied. The professional physical educator in any teaching-learning situation should be fully cognizant of the implications of the theory underlying the knowledge and skills being taught to students. The physical educator without good, professional preparation and a thorough understanding of human motion must rely upon a pragmatic approach to the teaching-coaching process. This type of physical educator must, of necessity, rely on a trial-and-error process until he finds "something which works." The starting point for this usually is his own past experience originally conveyed, most likely, by other pragmatic teachers who learned the same techniques from their teachers before them.

The best traditional practices for developing strength, muscular endurance, cardiovascular endurance, flexibility, and skill should be maintained. The professional physical educator is better equipped than the physical educator without a functional kinesiologic background to evaluate traditional training methods and techniques for conditioning and skill development and thus better knows what to discard and retain. Another major advantage of the well-prepared physical educator is his ability to evaluate new or unorthodox approaches to performance. Also, this individual is capable of analyzing conflicting ideas regarding the improvement of performance. The pragmatist is at a distinct disadvantage under these circumstances because he does not have a working knowledge of analytic kinesiology. Or, he is intellectually unwilling to analyze in detail. Thus, students under his direction are not challenged to reach their potentials because their potentials remain untapped or unknown.

The professional physical educator must know *what* he is trying to accomplish and *why* he is imposing specific demands upon students in his efforts to bring about favorable adaptations and improved performances in sport, exercise, or dance. (Logan and McKinney, 1965) A functional knowledge of kinesiologic theory contributes considerably to the teaching-learning process in physical education.

Selected Books and Articles

1. Amar, J. *The Human Motor.* New York: E. P. Dutton and Co., 1920.
2. Anderson, T. McClurg. *Human Kinetics and Analyzing Body Movements.* London: William Heinemann Medical Books, Ltd., 1951.
3. Aristotle. *Progression of Animals, IX.* Translated by E. S. Forster. Cambridge: Harvard University Press, 1945.
4. Barham, Jerry N., and Thomas, William L. *Anatomical Kinesiology: A Programmed Text.* New York: The Macmillan Company, 1969.

5. BASMAJIAN, J. V. *Muscles Alive. Their Functions Revealed By Electromyography.* Baltimore: The Williams & Wilkins Co., 1962.
6. BOURNE, G. H. B., ed. *The Structure and Function of Muscle.* New York: Academic Press, Inc., 1960.
7. BRAUN, G. L. "Kinesiology: From Aristotle to the Twentieth Century." *Research Quarterly* 12:163, March, 1941.
8. BROER, M. R. *Efficiency of Human Movement.* Philadelphia: W. B. Saunders Company, 1966.
9. ———. *An Introduction to Kinesiology.* Englewood Cliffs: Prentice-Hall, Inc., 1968.
10. BUNN, JOHN W. *Scientific Principles of Coaching.* Englewood Cliffs: Prentice-Hall, Inc., 1959.
11. COCHRAN, ALASTAIR, and STOBBS, JOHN. *The Search for the Perfect Swing.* New York: J. B. Lippincott Co., 1968.
12. COOPER, JOHN M., and GLASSOW, RUTH B. *Kinesiology.* St. Louis: The C. V. Mosby Co., 1968.
13. COUNCIL ON KINESIOLOGY OF THE PHYSICAL EDUCATION DIVISION, American Association for Health, Physical Education and Recreation. *Kinesiology Review—1968.* Washington, D. C.: N.E.A. Publications-Sales, 1968.
14. DEMPSTER, W. T. "The Anthropology of Body Action." *Annals of the New York Academy of Science* 63:574, 1955.
15. DUVALL, ELLEN NEALL. *Kinesiology: The Anatomy of Motion.* Englewood Cliffs: Prentice-Hall, Inc., 1959.
16. DYSON, GEOFFREY H. G. *The Mechanics of Athletics.* London: University of London Press, 1964.
17. FAY, TEMPLE. "The Origin of Human Movement." *American Journal of Psychiatry* 111:644, 1955.
18. GANSLEN, R. V., and HALL, K. G. *The Aerodynamics of Javelin Flight.* Fayetteville: University of Arkansas Press, 1960.
19. GANSLEN, R. V. *Mechanics of the Pole Vault.* St. Louis: John S. Swift Co., Inc., 1963.
20. GRANT, J. C. BOILEAU. *A Method of Anatomy.* Baltimore: The Williams & Wilkins Co., 1948.
21. GRAY, HENRY. *Anatomy of the Human Body.* Philadelphia: Lea & Febiger, 1959.
22. HELLEBRANDT, FRANCES A. "Living Anatomy." *Quest* 1:43-58, December, 1963.
23. HILL, A. V. *Muscular Movement in Man.* New York: McGraw-Hill, Inc., 1927.
24. HIRT, SUSANNE P., and OTHERS. "What Is Kinesiology?" *Physical Therapy Review* 35:419, 1955.
25. INTERNATIONAL ANATOMICAL NOMENCLATURE COMMITTEE. *Nomina Anatomica.* New York: Excerpta Medica Foundation, 1968.
26. JOHNSON, WARREN R., ed. *Science and Medicine of Exercise and Sports.* New York: Harper & Row, Publishers, 1960.
27. KLOPSTEG, PAUL E., and WILSON, PHILIP D., eds. *Human Limbs and Their Substitutes.* New York: McGraw-Hill Book Company, 1954.
28. KNOTT, MARGARET, and VOSS, DOROTHY E. *Proprioceptive Neuromuscular Facilitation.* 2nd ed. New York: Harper & Row, Publishers, 1968.
29. LIPOVETZ, F. J. *Basic Kinesiology.* Minneapolis: Burgess Publishing Co., 1952.

30. LOGAN, GENE A. *Adaptations of Muscular Activity*. Belmont: Wadsworth Publishing Co., Inc., 1964.
31. LOGAN, GENE A., and McKINNEY, WAYNE C. "How About Why?" *The Physical Educator* 22:63-64, December, 1965.
32. MAREY, ETIENNE, J. *Movement*. Translated by Eric Pritchard. London: William Heinemann, Ltd., 1895.
33. MASSEY, BENJAMIN H., and OTHERS. *The Kinesiology of Weight Lifting*. Dubuque: Wm. C. Brown Company Publishers, 1959.
34. METHENY, ELEANOR. *Body Dynamics*. New York: McGraw-Hill, Inc., 1952.
35. MORRIS, ROXIE. "Anatomy Study Guide." Mimeographed. Los Angeles: University of Southern California, 1960.
36. ———. *Correlation of Basic Sciences with Kinesiology*. New York: American Physical Therapy Association, 1955.
37. MORTON, D. J., and FULLER, D. D. *Human Locomotion and Body Form*. Baltimore: The Williams & Wilkins Co., 1952.
38. MORTON, DUDLEY J. *The Human Foot*. New York: Columbia University Press, 1935.
39. MUYBRIDGE, EADWEARD. *The Human Figure in Motion*. New York: Dover Publications, Inc., 1955.
40. PECK, STEPHEN ROGERS. *Atlas of Human Anatomy for the Artist*. New York: Oxford University Press, Inc., 1951.
41. RASCH, PHILIP J., and BURKE, ROGER K. *Kinesiology and Applied Anatomy*. Philadelphia: Lea & Febiger, 1967.
42. RODAHL, K., and HORVATH, S. M. *Muscle as a Tissue*. New York: McGraw-Hill, Inc., 1962.
43. ROYCE, JOSEPH. *Surface Anatomy*. Philadelphia: F. A. Davis Co., 1965.
44. SCOTT, M. GLADYS. *Analysis of Human Motion*. New York: Appleton-Century-Crofts, 1963.
45. STEINDLER, A. *Kinesiology of the Human Body Under Normal and Pathological Conditions*. Springfield: Charles C Thomas Publisher, 1955.
46. THOMPSON, CLEM W. *Kranz Manual of Kinesiology*. St. Louis: The C. V. Mosby Co., 1961.
47. TRICKER, R. A. R., and TRICKER, B. J. K. *The Science of Movement*. New York: American Elsevier Publishing Co., Inc., 1967.
48. WALLIS, EARL L., and LOGAN, GENE A. *Figure Improvement and Body Conditioning Through Exercise*. Englewood Cliffs: Prentice-Hall, Inc., 1964.
49. WELLS, KATHARINE F. *Kinesiology*. Philadelphia: W. B. Saunders Company, 1966.
50. WILLIAMS, M., and LISSNER, H. R. *Biomechanics of Human Motion*. Philadelphia: W. B. Saunders Company, 1962.

part one

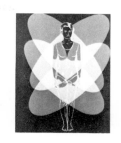

basic body movements and structures

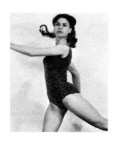

major joint movements

An understanding of motion as seen in sport, exercise, or dance has its basis in the knowledge of movements which are possible in the major joints (articulations) of the body. In analyzing skill, the following factors related to basic movements in joints should be known: (1) the type of joints involved, (2) the basic movements possible within these joints, and (3) the ranges of motion through which joints move during the performance. Movement occurs at joints as a result of muscles pulling on bony levers. The amount of motion possible within a joint is limited by the ligaments, other connective tissue, and bony structures.

▶ Classification of Joints

Joints are classified into three major categories: (1) synarthrodial, (2) amphiarthrodial, and (3) diarthrodial. When working with human motion, the first classification is not of any great consequence because *synarthrodial joints* are immovable joints, and they are relatively rare in the body. Examples of these are found in the sutures of the skull and in articulations between the teeth and mandible or maxilla.

Amphiarthrodial joints are those which allow a slight amount of motion to occur. There are two major subclassifications for amphiarthrodial joints. One is *syndesmosis*. A syndesmosis articulation is defined as two bones joined together by a ligament or an interosseous membrane. The bones may or may not touch each other at the actual joint. An example of this type of joint is the coracoclavicular joint. The other amphiarthrodial classification is known as *symphysis* or *synchondrosis*. This type of joint is typified by two bones joined together by a fibro-cartilage. The symphysis pubis is an example of this articular arrangement.

7

There are seven types of *diarthrodial*, or freely movable, joints. Each of these joints has a different type of bony arrangement within the joint. This is one factor which determines the motions possible by the joint: (1) *arthrodial* (gliding) joints consist of two plane, or flat, bony surfaces which butt against each other. There is very little motion possible in any one articulation of this type. More often, there is a series of arthrodial articulations which have the capacity to summate motion. Prime examples of these joints are found between the vertebral facets. This arrangement allows for flexion, extension, lateral flexion, diagonal flexion, diagonal extension, and rotation in the spine. (2) A *ginglymus* (hinge) joint is a uniaxial articulation, i. e., the articular surfaces of a hinge joint are shaped to allow motion in one plane only. An example of this type of joint is the elbow. The elbow allows flexion and extension only through the anteroposterior plane of motion while in the anatomic position. (3) A *trochoid* (pivot) joint is also a uniaxial articulation. One example, the atlantoaxial joint, has a bony pivot-like process which turns in a bony ring. Another example of a pivot joint is found at the proximal end of the radio-ulnar joint. (4) an *ellipsoid joint* is a biaxial ball-and-socket joint. It is ovoid in shape. An example of this type of joint is found at the articulations between the carpals and radius. The motions allowed within an ellipsoid joint are flexion, extension, abduction, and adduction. Any joint having the combination of these four movements also has a fifth movement, circumduction. (5) A *condyloid* (knuckle) joint is a biaxial articulation. It is also a ball-and-socket structure. One bone with an oval concave surface is received into another bone with an oval convex surface. Examples of a condyloid joint are found at the second, third, fourth, and fifth metacarpophalangeal joints. Flexion, extension, abduction, and adduction are the four basic motions allowed at the knuckle joints. The interphalangeal joints have the same bony configuration; however, the ligamentous structures surrounding the interphalangeal joints do not allow the joints to be abducted or adducted. Flexion and extension are the only motions possible within the interphalangeal joints. (6) An *enarthrodial* joint is a triaxial ball-and-socket joint. It is characterized by having a bony, rounded head received into a rounded, concave articular surface. A ball-and-socket joint of this type allows flexion, extension, abduction, adduction, diagonal abduction, diagonal adduction, and rotation. Rotation seen within an enarthrodial joint is around the longitudinal axis of the bone. Examples of enarthrodial joints are found at the hip and shoulder joints. (7) The *saddle joint* is a unique, triaxial joint. The carpometacarpal joint of the thumb is the sole example in the body. The two articulating surfaces at this joint are reciprocally concave and convex. This bony arrangement allows flexion, extension, abduction, adduction, and a slight amount of rotation within this joint. (Moore, 1949)

▶ Freely Movable Joint Structure

Since most motion is permitted at freely movable joints, an understanding of the structural components of a diarthrodial joint is necessary. The outer surfaces of the articulating bone are covered with a firm, smooth, and highly elastic material known as *hyaline cartilage*. This tissue is also called articular cartilage. Hyaline cartilage does not have a blood vascular network or nerves. As a result, there is very little, if any, ability for it to regenerate in case of injury. The hyaline cartilage serves three functions: (1) to absorb shock within the joint, (2) to smooth the articulating surfaces, and (3) to allow a greater freedom of motion within the joint by reducing the friction factor.

A freely movable joint has what is known as a *joint cavity*. It must be remembered that a joint cavity is a *potential* opening within the joint as opposed to a real opening. In a functional movable joint in a live human being, there is no appreciable space within the joint. A real joint cavity will appear within a joint when ligamentous and other connective structures surrounding the joint are elongated to their extreme, provided the surrounding musculature is relaxed. This condition may or may not be traumatic.

A freely movable joint has a sleevelike structure which serves as a "housing" for the joint. This is the *synovial membrane*. This vascular connective tissue completely surrounds the joint cavity. The synovial cells within the membrane secrete a viscous fluid known as synovial fluid. Thus, the major function of the synovial membrane is to provide joint lubrication. The synovial fluid also has a tendency to lubricate and nourish the hyaline cartilage.

Movable joints have an *articular capsule*. This is a fibrous structure or tissue surrounding the synovial membrane. The articular capsule functions, in part, to hold the articulating bones together. This capsule may be thought of as the outer "housing" of the joint because it has a direct relationship with stronger articulating structures known as the capsular ligaments.

Ligaments are integral parts of freely movable joints. They consist of fibrous tissue which reinforces the articular capsule. Ligaments hold bones together. Due to this function, ligaments serve as a major limiting factor to the degree of motion possible within freely movable joints. Ligaments must be stretched to improve flexibility.

Although ligaments regulate the extremes of joint motion, the muscles actually maintain the integrity of the joint. Strength of muscle groups surrounding a joint is directly proportional to the stability of a joint. Tendons are extensions of muscles as they cross most joints. As a result, one should not think of muscles and tendons as separate entities. A tendon serves to narrow the attachment of the muscle; consequently, the muscle will have a place at which to exert force on the bony lever.

A muscle belly and its tendon is one functional unit and will be discussed as such through this book.

▶ **Movement Nomenclature**

The inclusion of joint and body movement nomenclature into one's professional vocabulary is essential because an understanding of this terminology is one of the "working tools" of kinesiology. When undertaking an analysis of a performance, proper scientific terminology must be used to convey accurate information. Also, communication depends to a large extent upon accurate and consistent use of joint and body movement terminology.

When applying kinesiologic knowledge in the actual teaching situation, the instructor will find it necessary to communicate to individuals of different ages and varying academic backgrounds. For example, the tennis instructor may tell a student to "cock the wrist." To illustrate where confusion exists regarding this type of terminology, in tennis "cocking the wrist" usually implies radial flexion (Figure 2.1). In contrast, in badminton "cocking the wrist" may imply wrist hyperextension (Figure 2.2). Common terms or everyday language may be used functionally when teaching skills, but in conveying movement ideas to professional peers or in writing a kinesiologic analysis, scientific terms relating to movement must be used. The use of joint and body movement terms described below must become a part of the student's professional vocabulary. It is recommended that these terms be used in the teaching-coaching situation.

A paradox exists in regard to joint movements. Early anatomists used the anatomic position as the reference to describe human motion. In the anatomic position, the body is static and erect with the upper limbs extended at the sides and the palms of the hands face forward (Figure 2.3). Within the anatomic position there are three traditional planes of motion perpendicular to each other: (1) anteroposterior, (2) lateral, and (3) transverse. These planes of movement are discussed in detail in Chapter 3. Motions described by early anatomists were limited to these planes of motion. Difficulty arises when attempting to describe sport movements by using these three planes of motion exclusively. It is obvious in performing forceful or ballistic movements involving upper and lower limbs that there are diagonal movement patterns or planes of motion. To this time, no kinesiologists have attempted to describe diagonal planes of motion to facilitate communication in kinesiology. Owing to this, the concept of *diagonal planes* (Logan-McKinney diagonal planes of motion) is introduced in Chapter 3. The paradox mentioned above lies in the fact that *active joint movement* for *living*

Figure 2.1. Radial flexion.

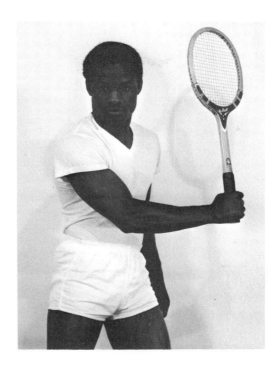

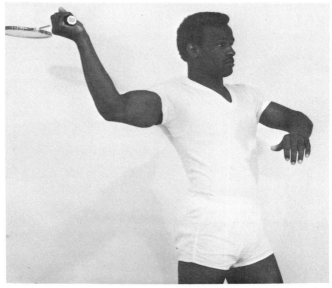

Figure 2.2. Wrist hyperextension.

individuals has been based in the past on *passive joint movement* of *cadavers*. (The anatomic position, anterior, posterior, and lateral views are shown in Figures 2.3, 2.4, and 2.5.) The anatomic position does serve as a reference point for the movements listed below. This is the main purpose of the anatomic position.

Abduction is movement of a body part or limb away from the midline of the body. There are some exceptions to this. These are described later in this chapter. An example of abduction is movement of the upper limb away from the side of the body through the lateral plane of motion.

Adduction is movement of a body part toward the midline of the body. There are also some exceptions to this, and these are discussed later in this chapter. An example of adduction is the return of the abducted upper limb to the anatomic position through the lateral plane of motion.

Circumduction is movement of a limb or body part in a manner which describes a cone. Circumduction involves a combination of four

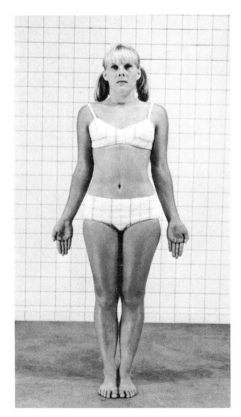

Figure 2.3. Anatomic position (anterior).

Figure 2.4. Anatomic position (posterior).

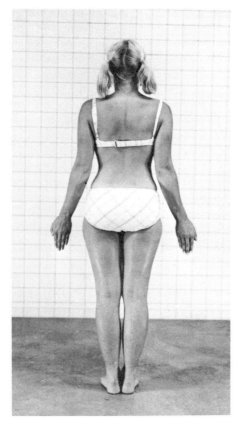

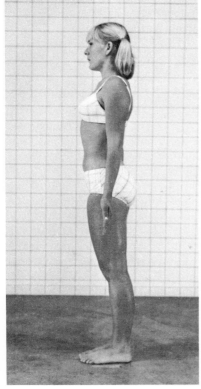

Figure 2.5. Anatomic position (lateral).

basic movements: (1) flexion, (2) extension, (3) abduction, and (4) adduction.

Depression is downward movement of the shoulder girdle. Very little depression within the shoulder girdle can occur from the anatomic position. Depression is the return movement of the shoulder girdle from elevation to the anatomic position.

Diagonal abduction is introduced as movement by a limb through a diagonal plane across and away from the midline of the body. An example of diagonal abduction at the shoulder joint is seen in the recovery phase of the back crawl swimming stroke (Figure 2.6).

Diagonal adduction is introduced as movement by a limb through a diagonal plane toward and across the midline of the body. An example for the upper limb would be the overhand throwing action commonly employed by the baseball pitcher. An example of hip joint diagonal adduction as employed by the punter in American football is seen in Figure 2.7.

Diagonal extension is a combination of rotation and extension of the vertebrae at the facets through a diagonal plane. This results in rib cage movement when the pelvic girdle is fixed or movement of the pelvic girdle when the rib cage is fixed.

Diagonal flexion is a combination of rotation and flexion of the vertebrae at the facets through a diagonal plane. This results in rib cage movement when the pelvic girdle is fixed or movement of the pelvic girdle when the rib cage is fixed.

Dorsiflexion is movement at the ankle joint of the "top" of the foot toward the lower limb, i. e., flexion of the ankle, or talocrural,

Figure 2.6. Diagonal   abduction—left shoulder joint.

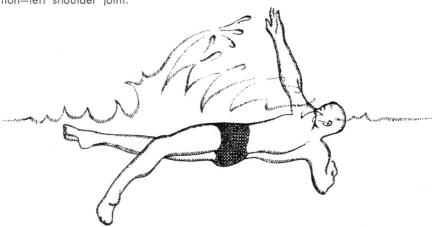

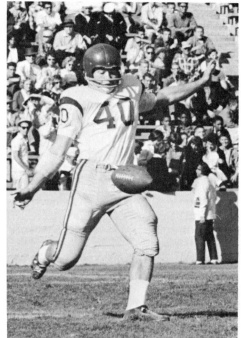

joint. Dorsiflexion action is observed in the sole of the foot trap used in soccer (Figure 2.8).

Elevation is upward movement of the shoulder girdle. The "shoulder shrug" is an example of this movement.

Eversion is movement of the sole of the foot outward. This movement takes place within the subtalar and transverse tarsal joints as opposed to the ankle joint.

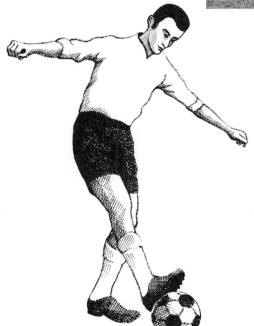

Figure 2.8. Right dorsiflexion.

Extension is any movement resulting in an *increase* of a joint angle. Most major joints are in extension while the individual is in the anatomic position. Complete extension of a body part approximates 180 degrees. For example, the elbow is extended while in the anatomic position when the entire upper limb is in a 180-degree position. (See Appendix C)

Flexion is any movement resulting in a *decrease* of a joint angle. For example, when the elbow is being flexed from the 180-degree extended position, the number of degrees within the joint angle is decreased as the hand moves toward the shoulder.

Horizontal abduction is movement of an upper limb through the transverse plane at shoulder level away from the midline of the body.

Horizontal adduction is movement of an upper limb through the transverse plane at shoulder level toward the midline of the body.

Hyperextension is movement of any joint beyond the joint's normal position of extension. Hyperextension of the cervical and lumbar spines, as an example, are seen during the swan dive. Hyperextension of the lumbar spine is seen in Figure 2.9.

Inversion is movement of the sole of the foot medially. If both feet are inverted, the soles of the feet will be toward each other. Inversion occurs at the subtalar and transverse tarsal joints.

Lateral flexion is movement of the head and/or trunk laterally away from the midline of the body. Lateral trunk flexion is seen when a gymnast performs a cartwheel.

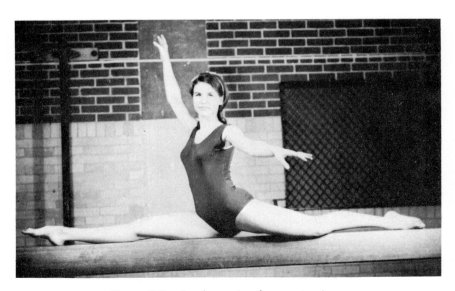

Figure 2.9. Lumbar spine hyperextension.

Opposition of the thumb is a diagonal movement of the thumb across the palmar surface of the hand to make contact with one of the four fingers. This thumb movement is commonly seen in gripping various sport implements such as golf clubs and baseball bats.

Plantar flexion is movement at the ankle joint of the sole of the foot downward. The term "plantar flexion" is an exception to the previous definition of flexion. In reality, plantar flexion is extension of the ankle. Most gross body movements in the vertical or erect body position begin with plantar flexion. Dancers use plantar flexion extensively for its aesthetic effect while performing (Figure 2.10).

Pronation is movement of the "back" of the hand forward. Pronation takes place at the radio-ulnar joint. When the hand is in a position of

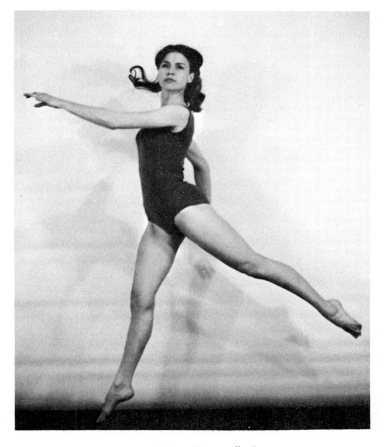

Figure 2.10. Plantar flexion.

pronation, the radius lies diagonally across the ulna. The hands, for example, are in a position of pronation while doing the push-up.

Prone position is the face-downward position by the entire body. The body does not have to be lying face downward on the ground or some other supportive surface. The prone position can be assumed, for example, in mid-air while rebound tumbling.

Radial flexion is movement at the wrist of the thumb side of the hand toward the forearm (Figure 2.1). As an example, the right wrist of the right-handed golfer is radially flexed during his backswing.

Rotation downward is rotary movement of the scapula with the inferior angle of the scapula moving medially and downward. The glenoid fossa is moved downward. Downward rotation of the scapula always accompanies adduction and extension at the shoulder joint. An example from sport of downward rotation of the scapula occurs during the pulling phase of the back crawl stroke in swimming.

Rotation laterally is movement around the longitudinal axis of a bone away from the midline of the body. Any overhand throwing or striking motion must include lateral rotation of the humerus. For example, lateral rotation of the humerus must take place prior to executing the overhead serve in volleyball, serving a tennis ball, or throwing a baseball. This action helps to place muscles on stretch.

Rotation medially is movement around the longitudinal axis of the bone toward the midline of the body. As an example, the "snap throw" of the baseball catcher involves medial rotation of the humerus immediately prior to the release of the ball.

Rotation upward is rotary movement of the scapula with the inferior angle moving laterally and upward. The glenoid fossa is being moved upward to accommodate the head of the humerus. Upward rotation of the scapula always accompanies abduction and flexion at the shoulder joint. An example from sport of upward rotation of the scapula occurs in basketball during the process of shooting the jump shot. The jump shot in basketball involves shoulder joint flexion; consequently, the scapula must be rotated upward.

Supination is the "palms forward" position of the hands in the anatomic position (Figure 2.3). Supination is the return movement from pronation, and it takes place at the radio-ulnar joint. When the hand is in a position of supination, the radius and ulna are parallel to each other. A flat handball serve involves a supinated hand.

Supine position is lying with the body in a face-up position. The body does not have to be lying face upward on a supportive surface. It may be suspended in air in a supine position. This is observed in diving and rebound tumbling.

Ulnar flexion is movement of the little finger side of the hand toward the forearm. Ulnar flexion in both wrists is seen at the point of impact in hitting a baseball or softball.

▶ Movement at Joints

Within this section there is a discussion of all movement within selected joints. Movements are illustrated for reference purposes. Arrows are included in the illustrations to indicate the direction of movement. See Appendix C for joint range of motion recording forms.

For organization and discussion purposes in this section and in Part 3, the discussion will proceed from the foot upward through the major joints of the body.

INTERPHALANGEAL JOINTS OF THE TOES—These joints are classified as condyloid joints. Due to the specialized nature of the ligamentous tissue surrounding these joints, flexion and extension are the only movements possible (Figure 2.11). The movement of flexion in the interphalangeal joints is through a range of 90 degrees. The toes are flexed from a starting or extended position of 180 degrees to a completely flexed position of 90 degrees. Extension is the return from flexion, i. e., the angle is increased from 90 degrees to 180 degrees. Some hyperextension may be observed at times within these joints, especially when attempting to maintain equilibrium.

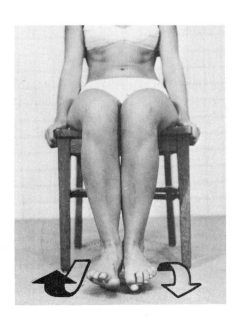

Figure 2.11. Interphalangeal joint movements.

METATARSOPHALANGEAL JOINTS. These joints are classified as condyloid. Movements allowed are flexion, extension, abduction, and adduction. Flexion and extension are seen in Figure 2.11. Ranges of motion are limited for abduction and adduction movements at these joints. Flexion occurs through a range of thirty-five degrees. Extension is possible through a range of eighty degrees; however, the last forty-five degrees of extension is more properly called hyperextension.

Although abduction and adduction of the toes are relatively minor movements within an analysis of a sport skill, the reference point for these movements should be noted. The reference line for abduction and adduction within the feet and hands differs from the abduction and adduction line for other body parts. Within the foot, the reference line for these movements runs longitudinally through the second toe.

TARSOMETATARSAL JOINTS. These arthrodial joints allow a small amount of gliding movement. The joints are located between the cuneiform bones, the cuboid and proximal ends of the five metatarsals.

TRANSVERSE TARSAL AND SUBTALAR JOINTS. These joints consist of the articulations between the talus and navicular bones as well as the calcaneus and cuboid bones. The movements of inversion and eversion take place within the subtalar and transverse tarsal joints (Figures 2.12 and 2.13). The movement possible between the talus and calcaneus supplements the movement of inversion and eversion. See Appendix A.

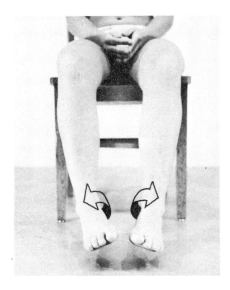

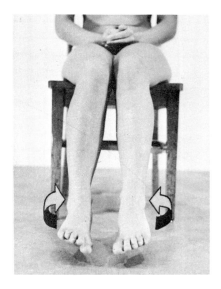

Figure 2.12. Inversion.   **Figure 2.13.** Eversion.

TALOCRURAL JOINT (ANKLE JOINT)—The bones involved at this joint are the tibia, fibula, and talus. This hinge joint allows dorsiflexion and plantar flexion only (Figure 2.14 and Figure 2.15). However, a slight amount of rotation may take place within the talocrural joint. Dorsiflexion occurs through approximately fifteen degrees, and plantar flexion takes place through approximately forty-five degrees.

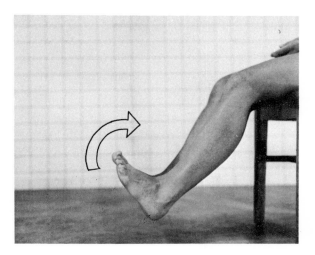

Figure 2.14. Dorsiflexion.

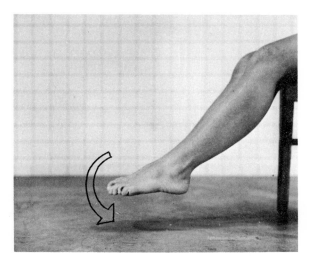

Figure 2.15. Plantar flexion.

KNEE JOINT—The bones involved at this joint are the femur, tibia, and patella. This joint is a trochoginglymus, or modified hinge, joint. It is so classified because the knee joint allows flexion (Figure 2.16), extension (Figure 2.17), and slight rotation medially (Figure 2.18) and laterally (Figure 2.19). The knee joints are in extension in the anatomic position. This is considered to be 180 degrees. The knee may be flexed through a range of 130 degrees. When the knee is flexed, slight medial and lateral rotations are possible.

Figure 2.16.   Knee flexion.

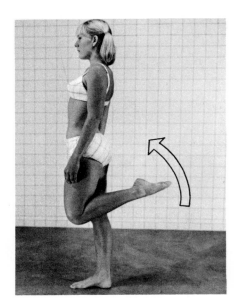

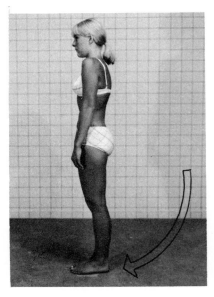

Figure 2.17.   Knee extension.

The patella is a sesamoid bone lying within the quadriceps femoris tendon. It must be remembered that the posterior surface of the patella has a cartilaginous surface which articulates with the femur. The patella serves two functions within this articulation: (1) protects the knee joint and (2) increases the angle of pull of the quadriceps femoris muscle group.

Figure 2.18. Medial rotation of the left knee.

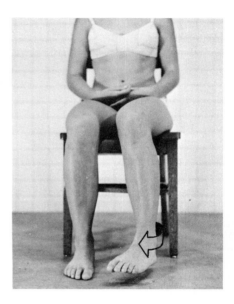

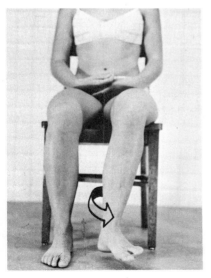

Figure 2.19. Lateral rotation of the left knee.

HIP JOINT—The bones involved at this joint are the pelvis and femur. Specifically, the hip joint consists of the articulation between the head of the femur and acetabulum. The hip joint is a ball-and-socket, or enarthrodial, joint. This joint allows flexion (Figure 2.20), extension

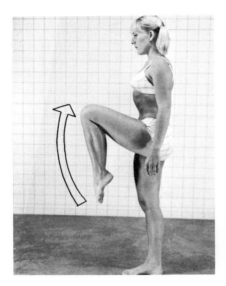

Figure 2.20. Hip flexion.

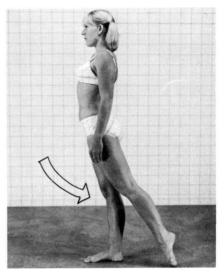

Figure 2.21. Hip extension.

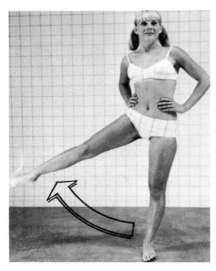

Figure 2.22. Hip abduction.

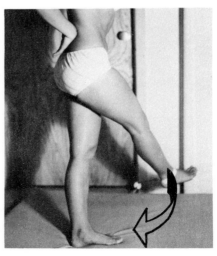

Figure 2.23. Diagonal abduction of the hip.

(Figure 2.21), abduction (Figure 2.22), adduction or the return from abduction to the anatomic position, diagonal abduction (Figure 2.23), diagonal adduction (Figure 2.24), medial rotation (Figure 2.25), and lateral rotation (Figure 2.26).

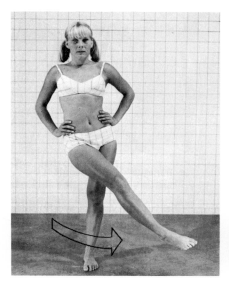

Figure 2.24. Diagonal adduction of the hip.

Figure 2.25. Medial rotation of the hip.

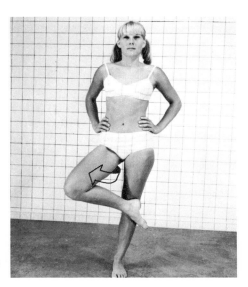

Figure 2.26. Lateral rotation of the hip.

Experience has indicated that confusion exists when discussing the hip. In common usage, many people use the term "hip" to refer to the iliac crests. The use of the term in this manner is not completely incorrect, because the iliac crests are parts of the hipbone, or pelvic girdle. However, the hip joint should never be confused with the entire pelvic girdle. Hip joint movements are of prime concern to the physical educator when analyzing performance. The iliac crests are also valuable anatomic landmarks while analyzing performers in sports, and they can be used extensively as such without confusion arising between iliac crest and hip joint movements.

The two major ball-and-socket joints of the body, the hip and shoulder joints, have similar motion. The amount of motion within these joints differs owing to their differing functions. The primary purposes of the hip joint are stability and weight bearing. The depth of the acetabulum in receiving the femoral head allows for these purposes. The depth of the glenoid fossa is relatively shallow when compared with the acetabulum; consequently, the shoulder joint permits greater ranges of motion than the hip joint. The ranges of motion seen at the shoulder joints allow performers to execute a wide variety of neuromuscular skills. Because of the required functions of the hip joint, however, the ranges of motion are relatively less than those found in the ball-and-socket joint at the shoulder.

The average range of motion for hip joint flexion is 125 degrees. Hip flexion is shown in Figure 2.20. It should be noted that the knee of the subject is also flexed in this illustration. If the knee were extended, the subject would be able to go through approximately 90 degrees of hip flexion only. Therefore, flexing the knee allows for an additional 35 degrees of hip flexion. This is the result of the mechanical and spatial arrangement of the muscles on the posterior aspects of the knee and hip joints.

Hip extension is merely the return movement from flexion to the anatomic position. Hip abduction (Figure 2.22) occurs through a range of approximately forty-five degrees. Adduction of the hip is the return from abduction to the anatomic position. Diagonal abduction of the hip is shown in Figure 2.23, and the extreme of diagonal adduction is shown in Figure 2.24. The range of motion for diagonal abduction at the hip is approximately sixty degrees. Diagonal adduction is the return movement through the diagonal plane of motion.

Rotary movements at the hip are around the longitudinal axis of the femur. The total, combined rotary action of the hip is ninety degrees. Medial rotation takes place through forty-five degrees of motion, and lateral rotation also occurs through forty-five degrees. Medial and lateral rotation at the hip joint starts from the anatomic position.

PELVIC GIRDLE MOVEMENTS—Although some terminology exists in the literature regarding pelvic girdle movement, it tends to be ambiguous and confusing. Thus, illustrative examples and new terminology for pelvic girdle movements are introduced. These are illustrated in Figures 2.27, 2.28, and 2.29. The purpose for presenting new pelvic girdle movement terminology is to provide for better communication in performance analyses. The iliac crests are the most important anatomic landmarks to observe for pelvic girdle movements. Pelvic girdle movements described are in relation to the three traditional planes of motion: (1) anteroposterior, (2) lateral, and (3) transverse. Although pelvic girdle movements can be described anatomically as a combination of movements taking place at the hip joint and/or lumbar spine, the terminology presented is in reference specifically to movement of the pelvic girdle *per se*.

Six pelvic girdle movements are introduced. Figure 2.27 shows the paired pelvic girdle movements in the transverse plane. The transverse plane is around the longitudinal axis of the body. As seen in the illustration, in the standing position *right transverse pelvic rotation* takes place clockwise, or to the performer's right, and *left transverse pelvic rotation* takes place counterclockwise, or to the performer's left. Baseball coaches often use the term "open the hips" as a coaching suggestion for hitters. For the right-handed hitter in baseball, "opening the hips" simply means a more pronounced left transverse rotation of the pelvic girdle during the movement phase of hitting.

Figure 2.27. Transverse pelvic girdle rotation. Arrows indicate direction of pelvic movement around a longitudinal axis (top view).

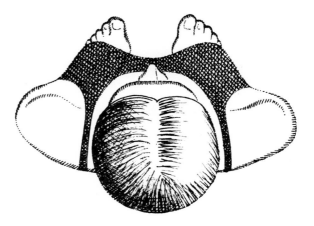

Figure 2.28 shows anteroposterior pelvic movement. The axis for the anteroposterior plane is lateral, i. e., from side to side. As stated previously, the anatomic landmark for all of these pelvic movements is the crest of the ilium. In *anterior pelvic rotation* the iliac crests move forward. Conversely, *posterior pelvic rotation* results in the iliac crests' being moved backward. An example of posterior pelvic girdle rotation is the so-called "bump action" of the burlesque dancer.

Lateral pelvic rotation is illustrated in Figure 2.29. Lateral pelvic rotation takes place either right or left through the lateral plane, and the axis is anteroposterior. It occurs unilaterally when the weight is borne either by the hands or on one leg. For example, right lateral rotation of the pelvic girdle takes place when the body weight is borne on the left leg while standing. The movement involves elevation of the right iliac crest. Since all of these movements are in relation to the pelvic girdle only, no degrees of motion are given.

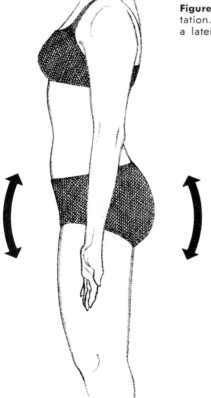

Figure 2.28. Anteroposterior pelvic girdle rotation. Arrows indicate pelvic movement around a lateral axis through hip joints.

Figure 2.29. Lateral pelvic girdle rotation. Arrows indicate pelvic movement around an anteroposterior axis through center of the pelvis.

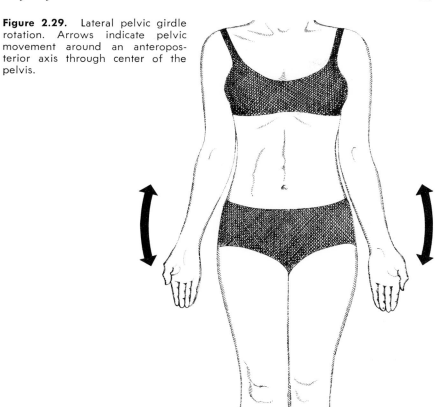

THE SPINAL COLUMN—Generally, most motion within the spinal column takes place in the lumbar and cervical regions. Although the total summation of movement within the spinal column appears great, there is relatively little motion between individual vertebrae.

For kinesiologic analyses, the spinal column is thought of as having three functional units: (1) the lumbar spine and pelvic girdle, (2) thoracic spine and rib cage, and (3) cervical spine and head. Contrary to traditional study of the spinal column in the anatomic position, it is essential in kinesiology that the spinal column be considered for study in the following positions or situations: (1) in a weight-bearing position on one or both feet, (2) with the weight being borne by the hands, (3) in a non-weight-bearing position, or (4) in the water.

Lumbar movement may initiate pelvic girdle movement or thoracic-rib cage movement. This is dependent upon which of these two body areas is fixed at a given time. For example, when the weight of the body is borne by the feet, an attempt to touch the toes with the fingertips results in lumbar flexion. The pelvic girdle remains relatively stable, and the moving part is the thoracic spine-rib cage. When hanging by the hands from a horizontal bar, lumbar flexion results in movement of the pelvic girdle, and the thoracic spine-rib cage remains relatively fixed. This is the opposite of the weight-bearing position when the weight is being borne by the feet. When unsupported, as in rebound tumbling, lumbar flexion would result in pelvic girdle movement or thoracic-rib cage movement depending upon which of these two body parts is most stable at any given time while the body is in free flight. The moving body segment is dependent upon the part serving as the axis of the body mass. This axis does change, for example, during the course of a rebound tumbling sequence.

Movements in the lumbar spine are as follows: Lumbar flexion is shown in Figure 2.30; Lumbar extension is simply the return from lumbar flexion to the anatomic position; Hyperextension of the lumbar spine is also possible (Figure 2.31); Lateral flexion of the lumbar spine (Figure 2.32) is described as being either right or left depending upon which side of the body is being flexed. *Lateral flexion of the lumbar spine is always accompanied by slight spinal rotation.* The normal spinal curve within the lumbar area is anteroposterior. When lateral flexion occurs in the lumbar spine, a lateral curve is induced. This superimpos-

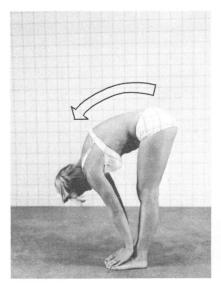
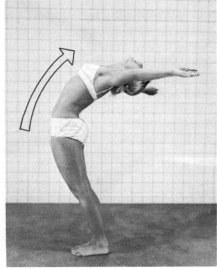

Figure 2.30. Lumbar flexion.   **Figure 2.31.** Lumbar hyperextension.

ing of a lateral curve on an anteroposterior curve causes rotation to take place within or between the vertebrae.

Spinal rotation is movement of the rib cage right or left in relation to the longitudinal axis of the body (Figure 2.33). Due to the bony arrangement of the lumbar spine, very little rotation actually occurs in this area. The two functional units, which include the pelvic girdle and lumbar spine as well as the thoracic spine and rib cage, move as a unit when the lumbar spine is flexed, extended, diagonally flexed, diagonally extended, laterally flexed, or rotated.

Figure 2.32. Lateral flexion (right).

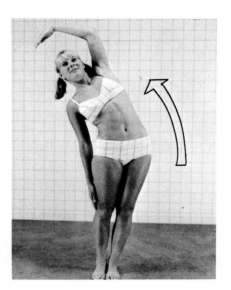

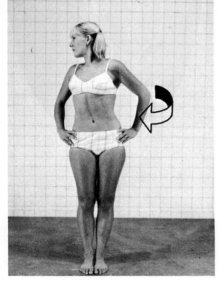

Figure 2.33. Spinal rotation (right).

The functional unit of the head and cervical spine permits a wide variety of movements. Cervical flexion (Figure 2.34) is movement of the head anteriorly. Extension is the return movement from flexion to the anatomic position. Hyperextension of the cervical spine is used frequently in sports (Figure 2.35). For example, the wrestler uses cervical spine hyperextension while "bridging." The football player who must block or tackle is taught by his coach to "keep his head up." "Keeping the head up" in this context is an example of cervical hyperextension. Lateral flexion of the cervical spine involves movement of the head to the right or left (Figure 2.36). Rotation of the cervical spine must occur with lateral flexion of the cervical spine. The same principles involving curves are involved here as in the previous discussion about the lumbar spine. Cervical spine rotation takes place around the longitudinal axis of the body (Figure 2.37). Cervical spine rotation is described as being either right or left depending upon the direction of movement of the head in relation to the individual's body. In rebound tumbling and diving, as examples, movements occurring in the functional unit of the cervical spine and head tend to initiate movements in other parts of the body. This, of course, has its basis in neurologic reflexes active in head and neck areas.

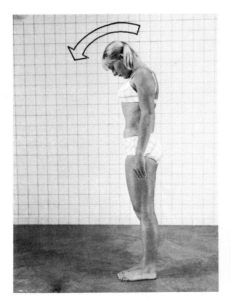
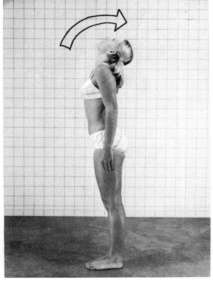

Figure 2.34. Cervical flexion.   **Figure 2.35.** Cervical hyperextension.

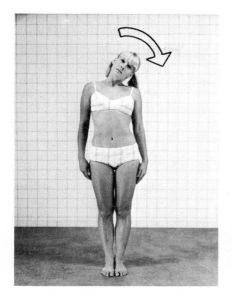 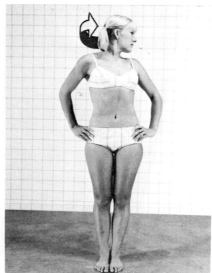

Figure 2.36. Lateral flexion (left) cervical spine.

Figure 2.37. Cervical rotation (left).

SHOULDER GIRDLE MOVEMENTS—A girdle is designed to encompass or encircle an area. The pelvic girdle is an example of a "true girdle," because the pelvic girdle is roughly an ovoid structure. In contrast, the shoulder girdle is not a complete ovoid structure composed of bone. The shoulder girdle is interrupted anteriorly and posteriorly. The clavicle is attached to the sternum anteriorly. Posteriorly, the scapula is attached to the spine by muscles. The interrelationship of bone and muscle in this area does form an ovoid-type structure.

The sternoclavicular joint is the most freely movable gliding joint in the body. Since the sternoclavicular joint is a part of the shoulder girdle and the scapulae are attached to the spine by muscles, there is a great amount of potential motion within the shoulder girdle. This is in direct contrast to the pelvic girdle which allows a relatively small amount of motion.

The moving bony parts of the shoulder girdle are the two scapulae and two clavicles. The articulation between each clavicle and scapula takes place at the acromioclavicular joint. During the many movements of the shoulder girdle, the spine of the scapula and the clavicle maintain approximately a forty-five-degree angle to each other. This constant relationship between the scapula and the clavicle is possible since very little motion is possible within the acromioclavicular joint. Functionally, the acromioclavicular joint could be a solid unit without the loss of too much motion within the shoulder girdle proper. Of the three joints involved in the shoulder area, the sternoclavicular and glenohumeral joints provide the greatest potential for motion.

For purposes of discussion, the shoulder girdle is considered separately. However, the shoulder girdle area and the shoulder joint must function in conjunction with each other in a "teamwork" manner. Movements of the shoulder joint usually involve scapular action. The reciprocal action between the humerus and the glenoid fossa of the scapula allows for a wide range of motion to take place within the glenohumeral joint. The scapula is also treated as a separate entity for discussion purposes. In reality, its total movement is integrated with clavicular and humerus movements.

In the shoulder area there are six scapular movements. Rotation of the clavicle is not included because it is relatively slight. It takes place around the longitudinal axis of the clavicle. When clavicular rotation does occur, the scapula is also moving owing to the fact that the acromioclavicular joint is a fixed joint. Scapular movements are as follows: (1) abduction (Figure 2.38), (2) adduction (Figure 2.39), (3) upward rotation (Figure 2.40), (4) downward rotation (Figure 2.41), (5) elevation (Figure 2.42), and (6) depression (Figure 2.43).

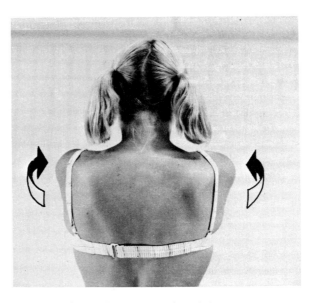

Figure 2.38. Scapular abduction.

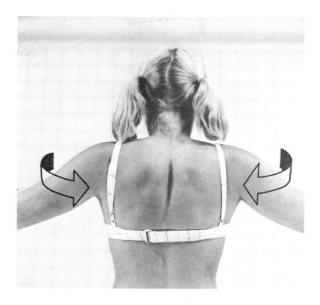

Figure 2.39.   Scapular adduction.

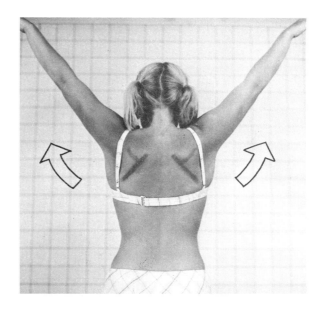

Figure 2.40.   Upward rotation of the scapulae.

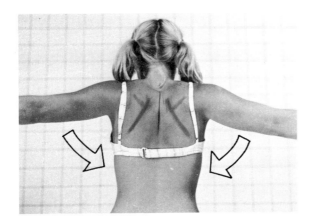

Figure 2.41.   Downward rotation of the scapulae.

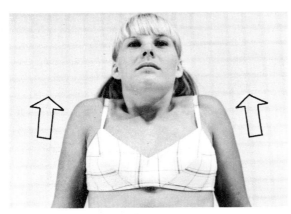

Figure 2.42.   Elevation.

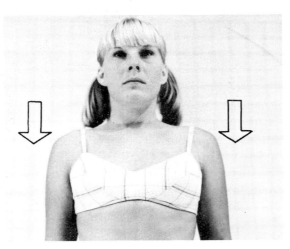

Figure 2.43.   Depression.

SHOULDER JOINT MOVEMENTS—As indicated above, any time motion occurs at the glenohumeral joint there is concomitant action within the shoulder joint; however, there is one skeletal deterrent which must be considered when discussing shoulder joint movements. To abduct the humerus through a 180-degree range while it is medially rotated is impossible. The humerus must first be laterally rotated to allow it to go through 180 degrees of shoulder joint abduction. Lateral rotation allows the head of the humerus to clear the inferior surface of the acromion process. This action involves a concept known as "force couple action," which will be discussed in detail in Part Two.

In addition to the eight shoulder joint movements found in the literature, two additional shoulder joint movements are introduced here and described. These are diagonal adduction (Figure 2.44) and diagonal abduction (Figure 2.6, p. 14). The introduction of these movements was deemed necessary because diagonal movement patterns are very common in sports performances. The eight traditional movements attributed to the shoulder joint are (1) abduction (Figure 2.45), (2) adduction is the return

Figure 2.44. Diagonal adduction of the right shoulder joint.

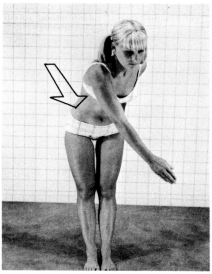

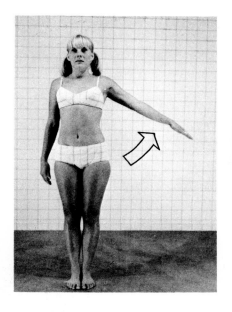

Figure 2.45. Shoulder joint abduction.

from abduction to the anatomic position, (3) flexion (Figure 2.46), (4) hyperextension (Figure 2.47), (5) horizontal abduction (Figure 2.48), (6) horizontal adduction is the return action from horizontal

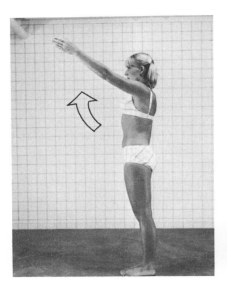

Figure 2.46.   Shoulder joint flexion.   **Figure 2.47.**   Shoulder joint hyperextension.

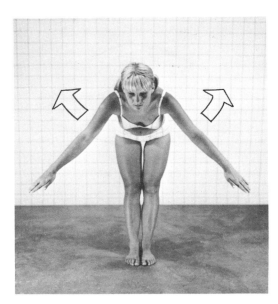

Figure 2.48.   Horizontal abduction of the shoulder joints.

abduction, (7) medial rotation (Figure 2.49), and (8) lateral rotation (Figure 2.50).

There are varying ranges of motion in the shoulder joint. Diagonal adduction takes place through approximately 200 degrees of motion, and diagonal abduction is simply the return from diagonal adduction. Abduction is possible through 180 degrees *if* the humerus is laterally rotated. Adduction is, of course, the return from abduction. Flexion at the shoulder joint occurs through a range of 180 degrees, and extension is the

Figure 2.49. Medial rotation of the right shoulder.

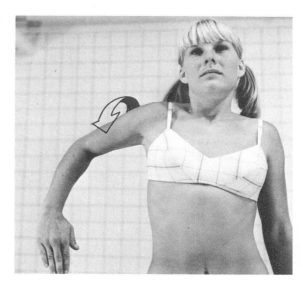

Figure 2.50. Lateral rotation of the right shoulder.

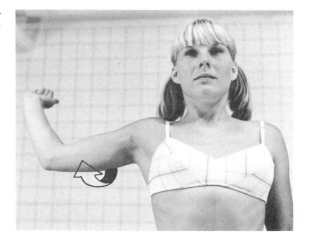

return from flexion. Horizontal adduction takes place through approximately 100 degrees, and horizontal abduction is the return action through the same range of motion. These two movements are not seen too often in sport. Medial rotation, which takes place along the longitudinal axis of the humerus, occurs through a range of 90 degrees. Lateral rotation of the humerus around its longitudinal axis also moves through 90 degrees. The total range of motion of the humerus in a rotary fashion around its longitudinal axis is 180 degrees.

ELBOW JOINT MOVEMENTS—The elbow is a hinge joint allowing flexion (Figure 2.51) and extension. In the anatomic position the elbow is in a position of 180 degrees of extension (Figure 2.3, p. 12). The elbow

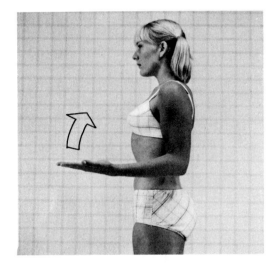

Figure 2.51. Elbow flexion.

of most individuals cannot go beyond the position of extension because of the bony projection at the proximal end of the ulna butting against the distal aspect of the humerus. Flexion of the elbow is mainly limited by the size or mass of the musculature on the anterior aspect of the upper limb. Flexion of the elbow takes place through approximately 150 degrees, and extension is the return from flexion.

RADIO-ULNAR JOINT MOVEMENT—Movements of the radio-ulnar joints result in supination (Figure 2.52) and pronation (Figure 2.53) of the hand. The hands are supinated in the anatomic position. If the hands are fully pronated from the anatomic position, they move through approximately 180 degrees. The return of the hands from a pronated position is supination. For purposes of kinesiologic analysis, the position of

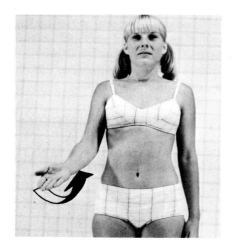

Figure 2.52. Supination.

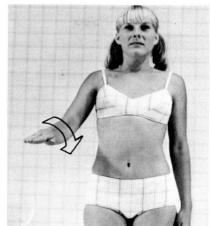

Figure 2.53. Pronation.

the elbow is very important in regard to pronation and supination. When the elbow is extended, medial and lateral rotation of the shoulder joint appears to pronate and supinate the hand. In order to be assured that supination and pronation are occurring in the radio-ulnar joints, the elbow should be at least slightly flexed. When the elbow is flexed, true pronation and supination occurs within the radio-ulnar joint.

WRIST JOINT MOVEMENTS—There are four movements possible at the wrist joint: (1) flexion (Figure 2.54), (2) hyperextension (Figure

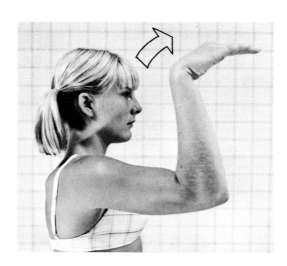

Figure 2.54. Wrist flexion.

2.55), (3) radial flexion (Figure 2.56), and (4) ulnar flexion (Figure 2.57). Flexion of the wrist takes place through approximately ninety degrees, and extension is the return from flexion to the anatomic position. Radial flexion takes place through twenty-five degrees. Ulnar flexion occurs through a range of approximately sixty degrees.

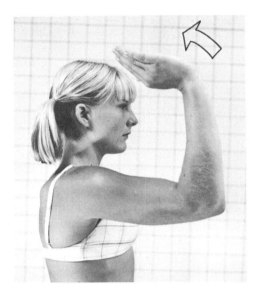

Figure 2.55. Wrist hyperextension.

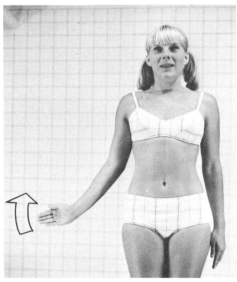

Figure 2.56. Radial flexion.

Figure 2.57. Ulnar flexion.

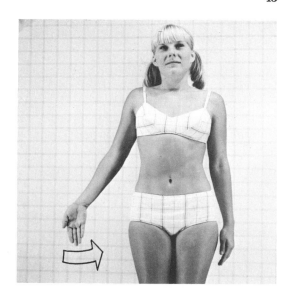

THUMB JOINT MOVEMENTS—There are three major joints to be considered in the thumb: (1) carpometacarpal (the saddle joint), (2) metacarpophalangeal, and (3) interphalangeal. The opposition action (Figure 2.58) is a unique function of the thumb. The motions possible within the saddle joint are flexion, extension, abduction, adduction, and a slight

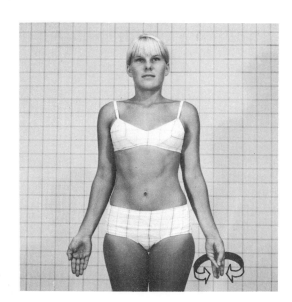

Figure 2.58. Opposition action of the thumb.

amount of rotation around the thumb's longitudinal axis. The thumb can move diagonally across the palm of the hand and work in opposition to any of the fingers. The metacarpophalangeal joint of the thumb allows flexion and extension. The interphalangeal joint of the thumb also allows flexion and extension only.

FINGER JOINT MOVEMENTS—The finger involves three major joints: (1) metacarpophalangeal, (2) proximal interphalangeal, and (3) distal interphalangeal. The metacarpophalangeal joints allow abduction and

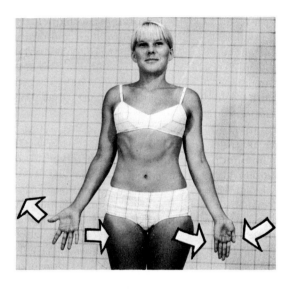

Figure 2.59. Finger abduction (right) and finger adduction (left).

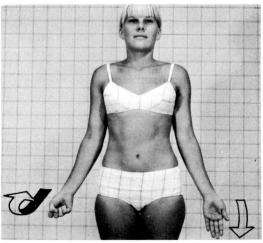

Figure 2.60. Finger flexion (right) and finger extension (left).

adduction (Figure 2.59) and flexion and extension (Figure 2.60). Each of the interphalangeal joints allows flexion and extension.

SELECTED REFERENCES

1. AHLBACK, SVEN, and LINDAHL, OLOR. "Saggital Mobility of the Hip Joint." *Acta Orthopaedica Scandinavica* 34:310-22, Fase. 4, 1964.
2. HIRT, SUSANNE P. "Joint Measurement." *American Journal of Occupational Therapy* 1:209-214, 1947.
3. MOORE, MARGARET LEE. "The Measurement of Joint Motion." *The Physical Therapy Review* 29:1-20, June, 1949.
4. MORRIS, ROXIE. *Anatomy Study Guide*. Mimeographed. Los Angeles: University of Southern California, 1960.
5. SALTER, N. "Methods of Measurement of Muscle and Joint Function." *Journal of Bone and Joint Surgery* 37-B:474-491, 1955.

planes of movement and selected anatomic landmarks

▶ Planes and Axes of Movement

For communication purposes, it is essential to have an understanding of the planes of movement. Briefly, a plane may be defined as an imaginary two-dimensional surface. To conceptualize a plane, it may be imagined as a windowpane without thickness dissecting an area of the body. Because of the structure of joints, the movement planes of motion for the human should be conceptualized as being oval in nature. The three traditional planes of movement—anteroposterior, lateral, and transverse—are shown in Figures 3.1, 3.2, and 3.3.

An axis of motion must always be considered with its plane of motion. An axis is an imaginary line through and perpendicular to a plane of motion. *Motion moving through a plane revolves around an axis.*

Historically, there have been three planes of movement described by anatomists. It must be understood that any movement of the body is in relationship to, and discussed in terms of, the plane of movement traversed. The first of the traditional planes is known as the anteroposterior plane. An example of a movement through an anteroposterior plane would be the hook-lying sit-up (Figure 3.4). This motion revolves around a lateral axis. The second of the traditional planes of movement is the lateral plane. The axis for the lateral plane is anteroposterior. An example of an exercise done in the lateral plane would be the "jumping jack" (Figure 3.5). The third traditional plane of movement is the transverse plane. The axis of motion for the transverse plane is parallel to the longitudinal axis of the body. Trunk or spinal rotation is an example of an exercise through the transverse plane of motion (Figure 3.6).

Many anatomists refer to horizontal and vertical planes of movement. Since these terms are related only to the surface of the earth, they tend

Figure 3.1. Anteroposterior plane of motion.

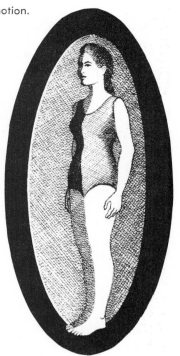

Figure 3.2. Lateral plane of motion.

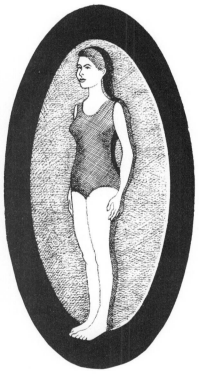

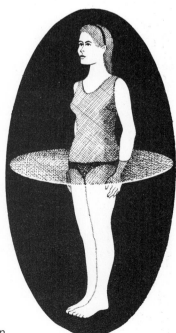

Figure 3.3. Transverse plane of motion.

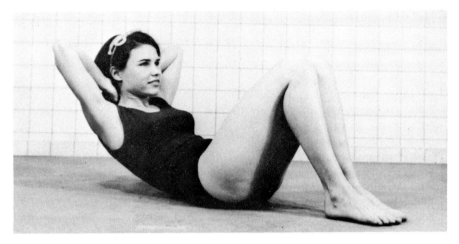

Figure 3.4. Hook-lying sit-up. A movement through the anteroposterior plane of motion.

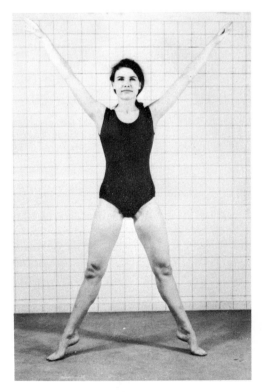

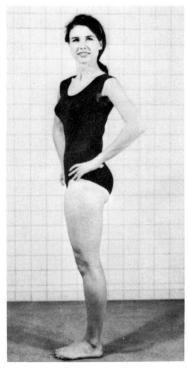

Figure 3.5. Jumping jack. A movement through the lateral plane of motion.

Figure 3.6. Spinal rotation. A movement through the transverse plane of motion.

to be misleading and confusing in regard to sport and movement. As an example, the transverse plane is a horizontal plane when the individual is in an upright position. The axis of motion in this example is vertical. Experience has indicated that confusion enters when the performer assumes a position other than the upright position. When the performer is lying supine, the transverse plane becomes a vertical plane, and the axis of motion is then horizontal. Therefore, the terms "horizontal" and "vertical" are not used herein to depict planes of motion because performers in sport, exercise, and dance are observed in a wide variety of positions in relation to the earth.

Although anatomic movements are named in relation to the trunk, the trunk need not be included in the movement through the plane of motion. For example, a one-arm biceps curl exercise involves elbow flexion and extension through an anteroposterior plane of motion with a lateral axis. The bench press is an example of an exercise done through the transverse plane with the axis longitudinal to the body. The overhead press is an example of an exercise done through the lateral plane with an anteroposterior axis.

Analyses of hundreds of sports skills have indicated that the traditional planes and axes of motion are inadequate for accurately describing sport performances. *Most ballistic sport skills are performed through planes of movement diagonal to the longitudinal axis of the body. Diagonal planes of motion* are described by the ranges of motion of the upper and lower limbs. The joints most involved in diagonal movement patterns are the hip and shoulder joints. Therefore, to add to the descriptive terminology for sports analyses, three new diagonal planes of motion are introduced as the *Logan-McKinney Diagonal Planes of Motion* to describe ballistic limb actions: (1) the *high diagonal* for upper limbs, (2) the *low diagonal* for upper limbs, and (3) the *low diagonal* for lower limbs. A high diagonal plane of motion of an upper limb is shown in Figure 3.7. The corresponding low diagonal plane of motion of the opposite upper limb is shown in the same illustration. A low diagonal plane of motion for the left lower limb is shown in Figure 3.8. Figure 3.9 is a composite of the diagonal planes. Figures 3.10, 3.11, and 3.12 illustrate athletes performing ballistic movement skills through the three diagonal planes of motion.

It should be noted that the traditional movements known as horizontal adduction and horizontal abduction are between high diagonal adduction and low diagonal adduction of the upper limbs through the transverse plane of motion. In practice, horizontal adduction and abduction are not used to a great extent in sports, especially when ballistic actions are an integral aspect of the skill. For example, a baseball hitter using these movements would always be hitting the ball out of his strike zone!

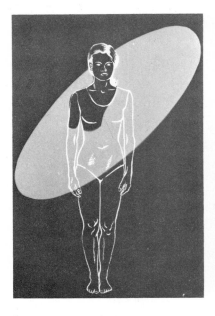

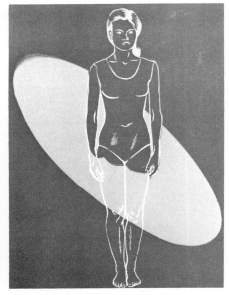

Figure 3.7. High diagonal plane of motion for the left shoulder joint.

Figure 3.8. Diagonal plane of motion for the left hip joint.

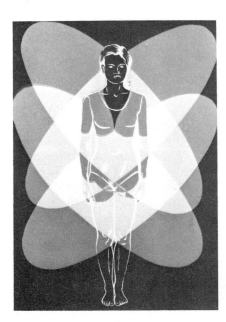

Figure 3.9. Composite of diagonal planes at both hip and shoulder joints.

Figure 3.10. High diagonal plane of motion as used by a left-handed pitcher.

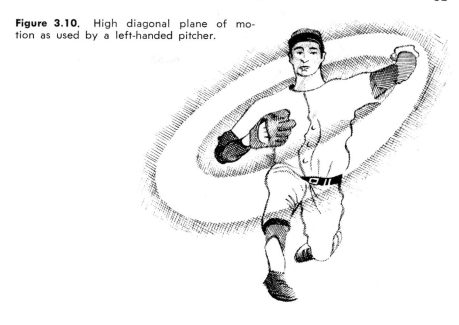

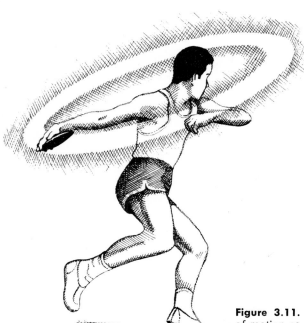

Figure 3.11. Low diagonal plane of motion as used by a discus thrower.

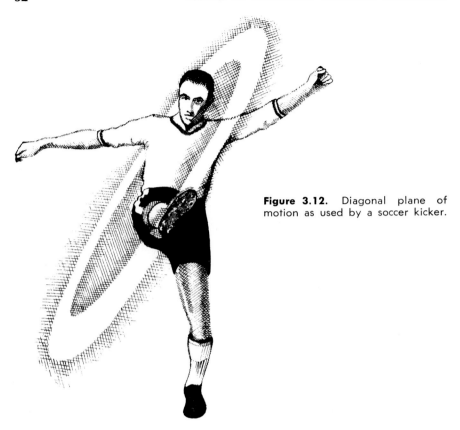

Figure 3.12. Diagonal plane of motion as used by a soccer kicker.

It is rather interesting to note that sports which tend to utilize the traditional planes of movement are the so-called "judged sports." Many times these sports, such as gymnastics, diving, and portions of weight lifting, have their bases for scoring in aesthetic factors. Perhaps there is a relationship between this type of activity and formal programs of physical education. Through 1927 the formal programs seen extensively in the past throughout Germany, Sweden, and in America had as their bases movement patterns associated with traditional planes of motion which were described by and borrowed from anatomists. It is rather obvious that calisthenics, wands, Indian clubs, and other activities of that nature were centered around the three traditional planes and axes of movements previously described. Many sport motions do not conform precisely to movement through the anteroposterior, lateral, and transverse planes of motion. On the other hand, calisthenics are easily adjusted to these planes, and this type of activity was, and is, seen in physical education programs.

▶ Selected Bones and Skeletal Landmarks

The assumption is made that a prerequisite course in human anatomy has been taken prior to undertaking a basic course in kinesiology. The introductory human anatomy course should include a detailed study of osteology and myology. Consequently, that subject matter is not repeated here in its entirety. However, a review of selected bones and skeletal landmarks is essential to understand the spatial relationship of muscles to joints.

A selected list of bones and skeletal landmarks appears in Figure 3.13. It must be stressed that this is a minimum list. These particular

FOOT	*Talus, calcaneus, navicular, cuboid, medial, lateral* and *intermediate cuneiforms,* tuberosity of fifth metatarsal, sustentaculum tali
LEG	*Fibula*—lateral malleolus, styloid process *Tibia*—medial malleolus, anterior border-medial surface, tibial tuberosity, medial and lateral condyles
THIGH	*Femur*—medial and lateral condyles, linea aspera, lesser trochanter, greater trochanter, head, neck
PELVIS	*Pelvis—Ilium, ischium, pubis*—pubic crest, crest of ilium, anterior and posterior, superior and inferior spines, ischial tuberosity, acetabulum
SPINE	*Vertebrae—cervical, thoracic, lumbar*—body, transverse and spinous processes—atlas and axis
CHEST	*Ribs, Sternum*—body, manubrium and xiphoid process
SHOULDER	*Scapula*—spine, acromion process, infra and supraglenoid tubercles, superior border, vertebral border, inferior angle, glenoid fossa, coracoid process, superior angle, subscapular fossa, supraspinatous fossa and infraspinatous fossa
ARM	*Humerus*—greater tubercle, lesser tubercle, head, anatomical neck, surgical neck, medial and lateral epicondyles, olecranon fossa, trochlea, capitulum, deltoid tuberosity, intertubercular groove
FOREARM	*Ulna*—olecranon process, coranoid process, styloid process, trochlear notch *Radius*—head, neck, radial tuberosity, styloid process
HEAD	*Skull*—mastoid process, zygomatic arch, mandible, maxilla, superior nuchal line, occipital protuberance.

Figure 3.13. Bones and skeletal landmarks. See Appendix A.

bones and skeletal landmarks were chosen because of their frequent usage in regard to the antigravity musculature and other major muscles of the body. Appendix A includes illustrations of these selected bones and skeletal landmarks.

These bones and skeletal landmarks are important for an understanding of the *spatial relationship of muscles to joints*. (Logan, 1964) The term "spatial relationship of a muscle to a joint" refers to the line of pull of the muscles between proximal and distal attachments as they cross a joint or joints.

Spatial relationship involves four knowledge factors. If known, they will enable the individual to *deduce muscle action*: (1) a knowledge of bone and skeletal landmarks to determine proximal and distal attachments of muscles, (2) the line of pull of the muscle as it crosses the joint which is determined by knowledge of the bony landmarks involved, (3) the movements possible within the joint or joints involved, and (4) the planes of motion through which the trunk or limbs move. If these four factors are known, action of a muscle group can be conceptualized and determined. For example, the middle fibers of the deltoid muscle attach distally at the deltoid tuberosity of the humerus. The proximal attachment is the acromion process of the scapula. This means that the muscle fibers of the middle deltoid must have a lateral spatial relationship to the shoulder joint. The shoulder joint permits all possible motions. Based on this information, what joint action would be seen in the shoulder joint if the middle deltoid muscle shortened, i. e., contracted concentrically? The deduced answer from the available evidence is shoulder joint abduction through the lateral plane of motion.

Rote memory is essential to learn initially the bones and selected skeletal landmarks. Also, rote memory is essential in the first stages of learning locations of muscles and motions possible within the joints of the body. Since kinesiology is a "working tool" of the physical educator, muscle actions, as a general rule, should be logically deduced from the information above rather than being memorized. This means that the physical educator must have a professional understanding of human motion. *Comprehension goes beyond memorization!* This method of studying the muscle action portion of kinesiology places the emphasis on conceptualization of muscle actions and joint movements. If accomplished, retention and subsequent use of kinesiologic theory in practice is infinitely more likely.

Selected References

1. HELLEBRANDT, F. A., and OTHERS. "The Location of the Cardinal Anatomical Orientation Planes Passing Through the Center of Gravity in Young Adult Women." *American Journal of Physiology* 121:465, 1938.

2. LOGAN, GENE A. *Adaptations of Muscular Activity.* Belmont: Wadsworth Publishing Co., Inc., 1964.
3. SWEARINGEN, J. J. "Determination of Centers of Gravity of Man." *Federal Aviation Agency Report* 62-14:37, August, 1962.

part two

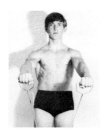

applied myology

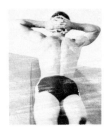

aggregate muscle action

Aggregate muscle action means that muscles work in groups rather than working independently to achieve a given joint action. This is a well-established scientific fact. (Taylor, 1931) In general, muscle groups must perform two major functions: (1) pull on bony levers to move the body and (2) maintain the body against the pull of gravity in a variety of positions both moving and stationary. Movement occurs in the body as a result of intricate teamwork among groups of muscles acting in a sequential fashion. Muscle action involves a complex series of sequential events, and muscle function during a given action may change rapidly. As an example, *muscles most involved* in initial movement will act on bony levers to perform a joint action during one phase of a skill. The same muscle group during a second phase of the same skill, however, will work to *guide* the bony lever a given distance. Toward the last part of the performance it is not uncommon to see the muscles which were originally most involved acting to *stabilize* a body segment so still another body part may move. Analyzing aggregate muscle actions is challenging due to such complexity of motion.

Knowledge of muscle functions has been derived in a variety of ways. Surface anatomy was probably the first source of study for people interested in anatomy. The term "muscle" was derived from the term "musculous," meaning "little mouse." This descriptive term was derived because some people thought the action of the bicep brachii shortening and lengthening during flexion and extension of the elbow seemed to depict a little mouse running up and down the upper arm immediately beneath the skin.

The study of muscle function through dissection techniques has only been in practice for approximately 600 years. The joints of cadavers were then moved through their ranges of motion in order to determine muscle actions. Such an examination of muscle action left much to be desired as indicated previously.

Another technique for studying muscle function is to study muscle action by omission. In certain pathologic conditions, such as poliomyelitis, some muscles become paralyzed and others remain normal. Observation of the loss of function at a given joint is an indicator of what the muscle does when it has its neurologic mechanisms intact in the normal individual. The major limitation in studying muscle action by omission is that normal musculature in the damaged area or near the damaged joint will have a tendency to substitute for the loss of function.

Palpation, determining the action of a muscle by the sense of touch, is another technique used in the past and also at the present time for determining muscle function. The major limitation of this technique is that the only muscles which can actually be palpated are the superficial muscles. However, this technique is recommended for the kinesiology student to help conceptualize the spatial relationship of superficial muscles to the joint involved for the motions under study.

The most accurate, but impractical, method of studying muscle function is by using electromyographic techniques. The electromyograph gives a direct reading of the amount and degree of muscle action potentials occurring during the contraction of a muscle. The electric muscle action potentials are received by electrodes either placed on the skin or implanted with needles within the muscle belly. Both of these electrode placement techniques limit the action of the performer in sport skills. Skin electrodes have a limitation of recording movement artifacts. This is unwanted information relayed into the oscilloscope or recorded on graph paper. Needle electrodes introduce a trauma factor into the performance. It is rather difficult to do an "all-out performance" with needles implanted in the muscles! Even with these limitations, electromyographic techniques are the most reliable to study muscle function, especially in the human performance laboratory situation.

▶ Neurologic Considerations

The central nervous system, like a computer, has several different levels which determine neuromuscular activity. These levels are the cerebral cortex, basal ganglia, cerebellum, brain stem, and spinal cord. Each of these areas has unique functions, and they all have integrative functions related to other parts within the central nervous system and the body as a whole. (Ayers, 1961)

The cortex is the highest level for integration of neuromuscular activity. The cortex is the area where volitional or willed movements are planned and initiated. Also, the cortex is the area where movement patterns can be inhibited. It must be remembered that the brain does not isolate individual muscles. Volitional movements are interpreted at the cortical level as aggregate muscle actions or patterns. Another important function of the cortex is the interpretation of sensory stimuli coming into the body via the various sensory organs. This very important function of interpretation of external and internal sensory stimuli is done in conjunction with the basal ganglia.

The basal ganglia are masses of gray matter within the cerebrum. They serve as "storage banks for data." Working in conjunction with the cerebral cortex, the basal ganglia can initiate gross, voluntary, *learned* movements. When movements or skills have been learned to the point that conscious thought is no longer needed, the basal ganglia will initiate movement patterns. The basal ganglia also provide a foundation for various postures and muscle tone. It is from this function that cortically directed movement can occur. The basal ganglia provide a balancing force for excitatory and inhibitory influences of the brain. There is control of the amount and intensity of the number of neurons working during muscle contractions. Another vital function of the basal ganglia is to control gross, rhythmic movements. Virtually all sport skills and movement patterns have a rhythmic aspect.

The cerebellum is the major integrator of sensory impulses in the brain. It integrates impulses from all sensory receptors and helps to modulate motor activity initiated elsewhere within the central nervous system. The cerebellum can be thought of as the "control center of the computer." The cerebellum is one area of the body which helps to control equilibrium. Along with this function it serves a related objective in that it also controls minute errors in relation to time and distance in movement. Although it controls these factors and acts as an integrator of all sensory stimuli, the cerebellum cannot initiate movements.

The brain stem integrates all central nervous system activity through excitation and inhibition of desired neuromuscular functions. Another major function of the brain stem is to control the postural tone of antigravity musculature. It must be remembered that well-conditioned antigravity muscles serve as the "foundation" for skilled performances. This concept will be discussed in Chapter 8. The brain stem is also vital because it activates the cerebrum which serves to help the individual maintain a wakeful state. The cerebrum also helps maintain an attention span, or concentration period, on a task for relatively long periods of time. These factors are all vital to high-level performance.

The spinal cord is simply a common pathway for all neuromechanisms related to the central nervous system. It integrates the various simple and complex spinal reflexes. In addition, it also integrates cortical and basal ganglia activity with the various classifications of spinal reflexes.

Voluntary muscle movements are the result of a complex relationship between the muscular and central nervous systems. Muscular movement patterns are initiated at various levels within the central nervous system. The quality of movement, in part, is dependent upon the neurologic information fed back from proprioceptors within muscles and joints to the higher brain centers. This information returning to the central nervous system from the periphery includes "data" concerning tension of muscle fibers, joint angles, and position of the body part being moved. This is analogous to computer systems now in use involving electronic servomechanisms. Thus, volitional movement is autoregulatory.

One of the major purposes of training is to assist the athlete in refinement of the neuromuscular integrative functions related to sensory information "fed into" the central nervous system. This information is coming from the eyes, ears, nose, skin, joints, and muscles. The proprioceptors located within muscles, and particularly within joints, are of vital importance to skilled performance. A few examples of these important muscle and joint proprioceptors are the intrafusal fibers or muscle spindles, Golgi tendon organs, and Pacinian corpuscles. These proprioceptors literally inform the central nervous system regarding the degree of tension within contracting muscle and the amount of movement taking place within the joints of the body during movements.

The neurophysiology of exercise is beyond the scope of this book. These basic neurologic concepts and neural functions are presented here to indicate that a sophisticated relationship does exist between the muscular and central nervous systems in regard to motion. A more detailed study of this interrelationship is indicated in a basic physiology course and in exercise physiology.

Traditionally, it has been common practice in kinesiology to present and study muscles and their actions on an individual basis. There is merit in this approach initially, but it does have its limitations. The major limitation is that muscles perform actions in an aggregate or group fashion. It has long been known that only group muscle actions are represented neurologically within the central nervous system. From a practical standpoint, the physical educator on the athletic field must analyze sport skill being performed by looking primarily at joint or body segment actions. After this has been done, he can deduce the aggregate muscle actions if he has a thorough understanding of kinesiology. It would be impractical and erroneous for the physical educator to think only in terms of individual muscle action.

▶ Sequential Muscle Action and Muscle Contraction

The specific function of a muscle is to develop tension or internal force. Movement occurs due to changes in tension within muscle groups acting on the bony levers. There are two forms of muscle contraction: (1) *isometric* and (2) *isotonic*. Isometric contraction is static contraction. No change in length takes place within the contracting muscles. As a result, no movement occurs within a joint. Isotonic contraction involves both shortening and lengthening of the muscle fibers. *Concentric contraction* takes place when the muscle is shortened, and *eccentric contraction* occurs when the muscle is lengthened. For example, when a thirty-five-pound dumbbell is held in the hand of an individual while standing and the elbow is flexed to 90 degrees from 180 degrees of extension, this is *concentric contraction* within the elbow flexors (Figure 4.1). When enough internal force is generated within the elbow flexors to maintain the 90-degree angle without movement at the elbow joint, this is *isometric* or *static contraction*. When more internal force is generated within the elbow flexors, the resistance of the weight will be overcome. The elbow will continue to flex to its extreme within the flexion range of

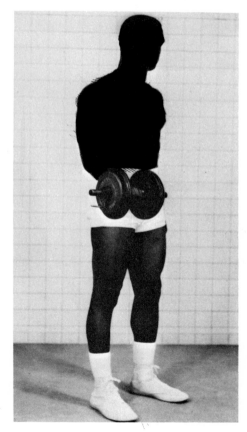

Figure 4.1. Concentric contraction of the muscles most involved for elbow flexion.

motion. This is concentric contraction, i.e., the elbow flexors have been shortened once more. If tension is decreased within the elbow flexors, the resistance of the thirty-five-pound weight will cause the elbow to be extended. This is an example of *eccentric* or *lengthening contraction* of the elbow flexors. Gravitational force would move the elbow back into extension in this example.

How does a muscle group contract? *A muscle tends to pull equally from its proximal and distal attachments toward its center.* For movement to occur within a joint at either end of the muscle group contracting, the other end must be stabilized momentarily. The range through which a muscle can change its length is known as its *amplitude*. This variation in length develops from a change of tension or shortening within the muscle, and this is concentric contraction. The release of tension allows the muscle group to lengthen—this is eccentric contraction. It is the production and release of muscle tension which produces joint movement. When a muscle elongates, it allows a bony lever or body part to move due to the pull of another muscle group, external forces, or the force of gravity. An elongating muscle group does not push a bony lever or body part.

In general, muscle groups work in pairs. When a muscle group contracts concentrically on one side of a body part, the muscle group on the opposite, or *contralateral,* side must lengthen. When the muscle group is lengthening on the contralateral side, it may or may not be under tension. The amount of tension present is dependent upon either the speed of movement of the limb or the amount of resistance overcome during the performance of the skill. If the muscular action must be repeated within the next fraction of a second, there are times when muscle tension cannot be found in either the shortening or lengthening muscle groups on either side of the limb. This is seen in the reciprocal ballistic leg movements of the sprinter. This cooperation among muscle groups is due to reciprocal innervation. (Sherrington, 1955)

During a slow movement, innervation produces tension within the muscle. This tends to be continuous within the muscle group contracting concentrically. In the lengthening contralateral muscle group, there is a relatively small amount of innervation and concurrent tension occurring, provided the slow-moving limb is not overcoming a resistance. When a muscle is lengthened, the stretch receptors within the muscles tend to be stimulated. When concentric contraction occurs within one muscle group on one side of a limb, there is an automatic neural action occurring to dampen the stretch reflex within the muscle group on the contralateral side of a limb. This is known as inhibition. When a muscle group is contracting slowly in a concentric fashion against a heavy resistance, the muscle group on the contralateral side of the limb may be under tension during the eccentric contraction of that muscle group.

When both muscle groups on either side of a joint are under tension performing a joint action at a very slow speed against great resistance, they are performing cocontraction. (Levine and Kabat, 1952) Two of the major purposes of cocontraction of muscles are (1) to protect the joint from trauma and (2) to stabilize joints or body parts.

The innervation sequence of muscle groups differs considerably between slow and fast or *ballistic muscle actions*. (Hubbard, 1960) Ballistic action is fast movement of a body part or limb through a range of motion assisted in part or wholly by momentum of that part through the range of motion. Ballistic movements are seen most commonly during alternating or reciprocal movements of the limbs. Movements of the upper and lower limbs in running are examples of ballistic muscle actions. Ballistic movements are also seen in sport skills involving transfer of momentum from one body part to another body part. They are vital in many sport skills where the kinesiologic construct of summation of internal forces is vital. Kinesiologic constructs are discussed in Chapter 10.

A ballistic movement is started by muscle contraction within a muscle group most involved for moving a joint. At the time of concentric contraction within this muscle group, there is concurrent lessening of muscle tension of the contralateral musculature. The concentric contraction starts the body part or limb into motion. When momentum takes over, there is a general cessation of electric muscle action potentials within the muscles most involved *and* the contralateral musculature. In other words, at this point in time, the limb is moving through its plane of motion without benefit of active contraction in either muscle group. The limb continues to move freely through its range of motion. Prior to reaching the end of the range of movement, innervation occurs within the contralateral musculature to slow the moving body part *and* provide the muscular tension or internal force necessary to move the body part in the opposite direction. It must be remembered that this burst of muscle tension occurs while the contralateral muscle group is contracting eccentrically. The "kick-back action" by the contralateral muscles occurs while the original muscles most involved for the joint action are devoid of tension. The original muscles most involved continue to remain devoid of tension until they are required to perform a "kick-back action" at the other end of the range of motion in a reciprocal or alternating action. Ballistic movement, with its "free-running phase," provides human beings with a high degree of conservation of energy during such activities as walking, running, and participation in a wide variety of sport skills. Without this neuromuscular mechanism, the individual would be unable to sustain muscular activity for prolonged periods of time.

To illustrate reciprocal ballistic movements, the following example is provided. With the arm flexed to ninety degrees at the shoulder joint, and the humerus medially rotated at the shoulder joint to allow flexion and extension of the elbow through the transverse plane, concentric contraction is initiated in the elbow flexors to provide a fast or ballistic movement of the forearm. Following the initial concentric contraction by the elbow flexors, the forearm moves through its range of motion by the momentum provided from the original burst of muscle contraction. The forearm continues to move rapidly through this range of motion until it is slowed when the action is reversed by eccentric contraction within the contralateral muscle group, the elbow extensors. The eccentric contraction of the elbow extensors occurs *before* the forearm has moved through the complete range of motion for elbow flexion. Once the eccentric contraction occurs within the contralateral muscles and elbow extension commences, there is a lessening of tension within the elbow extensors *and* flexors. The elbow continues to move into extension by momentum. Momentum is checked or slowed by the elbow flexors at a point near the end of the extension range of motion. This is done when the elbow flexors contract eccentrically to slow the motion and "kick" the forearm back into flexion. Once elbow flexion starts again, the above process is repeated. It can be seen that ballistic muscle action serves two purposes: (1) to perform reciprocal or alternating fast joint movements without wasted energy expenditure and (2) to protect the integrity of the joint.

All throwing and kicking actions are ballistic in nature, but they are not continuously reciprocal in nature. Ballistic action does protect the joints involved at the start and conclusion of the motion. For example, during baseball pitching, force is transferred from the trunk to the shoulder area just prior to diagonal adduction of the upper throwing limb. Timed with this force from the trunk musculature is a forceful burst of muscle contraction by the muscles most involved for diagonal adduction and medial rotation of the pitcher's upper limb. This sets the throwing limb into diagonal adduction. Once diagonal adduction has been started, the muscles most involved become devoid of tension. Momentum, augmented by the downward pull of gravity, moves the upper limb through diagonal adduction at the shoulder joint. This force is then transferred to the extending elbow. Just prior to complete elbow extension, diagonal adduction, and medial rotation of the shoulder joint, the elbow flexors and diagonal abductors contract eccentrically to slow the motion and ultimately stop the action. These very important eccentric contractions by the elbow flexors and shoulder joint diagonal abductors serve to protect the pitcher's elbow and shoulder joints.

It has been observed that throwing too hard during the early season causes pain in the back of the shoulder. This is the result of unaccustomed stress on unconditioned musculature, mainly the long head of the triceps brachii, which is used to stop the ballistic action of throwing.

As mentioned above, ballistic action conserves energy because there are phases within ballistic movements in which no muscle actions are being performed. A further conservation of energy occurs within the body owing to the action of two-joint muscles. Biarticular, or two-joint, muscles have attachments which cross joints at their proximal and distal ends. Biarticular muscles receive kinetic energy through momentum at one of their joints. This energy is subsequently utilized at the other joint. On the other hand, a one-joint muscle would lose this energy by dissipating it as heat.

There tends to be a mechanical advantage of a biarticular muscle over a uniarticular muscle, especially in the lower limbs. It conserves energy, particularly in biarticular muscles capable of flexing at one joint and extending at their other joint. Generally, the individual tends to flex and extend alternately within the hip, knee, and ankle joints during walking, jogging, and running. It should be remembered that muscles exert force in relation to their length. As the muscle shortens, its ability to exert force decreases proportionately. For example, when a basketball player jumps to rebound, he plantar flexes the ankle and extends the knee and hip joints. The biarticular muscle involved in the action at the ankle and knee joints is the gastrocnemius. During plantar flexion and subsequent knee extension, the gastrocnemius tends to maintain a constant length. *Flexion at one joint and extension at the second joint by a biarticular muscle results in a constant length. This allows it to exert a greater force throughout the action than if it were shortened at one end only.*

Other important biarticular muscles within the lower limb are the semitendinosus, semimembranosus, biceps femoris, rectus femoris, sartorius, and gracilis. When biarticular muscles are functioning on opposite sides of a limb, a greater force potential is present than when one-joint muscles perform the same function. In general, biarticular muscles work in an aggregate fashion with a strong uniarticular muscle at either end entering into the motion.

▶ Muscle Action Terminology

The muscles which overcome resistance and move a joint through a specified plane of motion are called the *muscles MOST involved* (MMI). (Wallis and Logan, 1964) The muscles most involved are located in relation to the joint so their line of pull lies parallel to or within the plane of motion through which the body part will travel. The term "muscles *most* involved" is a descriptive term designed for utilization with the concept of learning muscle action through use of knowledge regarding the spatial relationship of muscles to joints. This new term replaces such terms as "agonists," "prime movers," and "assistant movers." This should be remembered when studying other kinesiology materials.

The muscles located on the opposite side of the joint or body part from the muscles most involved are called the *contralateral muscles.* This term replaces "antagonists." The term "contralateral" indicates *location* of the muscle group. It *does not* indicate function. This was a limitation of the term "antagonists," because it implied that the antagonistic muscle group was *working against* the muscles most involved. As already discussed, contralateral muscles function in a teamwork fashion to perform motion *with* the muscles most involved.

Muscles are located on either side of the muscles most involved and the contralateral musculature and these are called the *guiding muscles.* These muscles help to rule out undesired actions. The descriptive term, "guiding muscles," replaces the terms, "helping synergy," "true synergy," and "synergistic action."

Muscles which hold a joint or body part to enable other body parts or joints to move are known as *stabilizing muscles.* This term replaces the term "fixator." Stabilizing muscles may be immediately adjacent to the moving joint or body part. They may also be remote from the moving body area. (Razumora and Frank, 1961)

A standard list of muscle actions, as seen in Appendix B, is limited. Such a discussion of muscle action does not consider effects on the human body of gravity and a variety of external and internal forces always acting upon the human organism. Historically, anatomists and kinesiologists have used the terms "agonists," "antagonists," "synergists," and "fixators" to describe muscular action. These terms are lacking as descriptive terms for muscle actions because they have been used in a context which has not taken into consideration the effects of gravity as well as as other external forces acting upon and within the body. There appears to be a need for change in terminology in this area. Consequently, within the book in hand kinesiologic terminology has been introduced which is believed to be more functional and descriptive.

The force of gravity, air resistance, friction, and other external forces must be considered when a given joint action takes place, especially when considering the muscles most involved for determining the extent and degree of motion at a joint. For example, reference to Appendix B will indicate that the muscles most involved in knee flexion are the semitendinosus, semimembranosus, biceps femoris, and gastrocnemius. This is true *if* resistance must be overcome, but there are situations where these muscles *would not* be the muscles most involved in controlling the extent of knee flexion. Such a case occurs when performing half-knee flexion from a standing position. The effect of the force of gravity must be considered because the mass of the body is being lowered primarily by gravitational pull. Consequently, the muscles most involved in controlling the extent or degree of knee flexion would be the quadriceps femoris muscle group on the anterior aspect of the thigh. The quadriceps femoris muscle group is actually controlling the amount or degree of knee flexion by contracting eccentrically. The hamstrings, which are traditionally described as knee flexors, are acting as contralateral muscles in this case. Therefore, there is seen a reversal of muscle function by these two muscle groups due to the effect of gravity.

Another example will help to illustrate the effect of gravity upon the muscles most involved for a given joint action. In the first example above it was noted that the body was being lowered in the direction of gravitational pull. What would happen to the muscle groups involved if the knee were flexed against gravity? With the individual standing on the right foot only, he is asked to flex the left knee through its full range of motion. Which muscles would be most involved for knee flexion? The answer is the "hamstring" muscle group because they are moving the knee through a range of flexion *against* resistance caused by the pull of gravity and the weight of the lower leg. The contralateral muscles in this case, i. e., the muscles which are eccentrically contracting, are the muscles within the quadriceps femoris group on the anterior aspect of the thigh.

The reversal of muscle action by muscle groups is seen when the body receives other external forces. For example, consider the elbow action of a catcher who is receiving a pitch delivered by a pitcher who can throw exceedingly fast. At the time of contact by the ball with the mitt, the elbows start through their range of flexion to absorb the impact of the ball, or the external force. Reference to the muscle list in Appendix B indicates that elbow flexion is done mainly by the biceps brachii, brachialis, and brachioradialis muscles. This would lead one to believe that these are the muscles most involved in this example because elbow flexion is occurring. On the contrary, the muscles most involved for elbow flexion in this example are the triceps brachii and anconeus muscles acting eccentrically at the elbow joint. The elbow flexors are acting as the contralateral muscles. The catcher's elbow is being forced into flexion for the most part by the external force created by the ball striking the mitt. The muscles most involved, triceps brachii and anconeus, are "braking the action," i. e., protecting the elbow joint and determining the degree of elbow flexion.

A thorough understanding of the reversal of muscle action caused by gravitational pull on the human organism is essential for kinesiologic analyses. It is especially important in the proper analysis and application of conditioning exercises for athletics and figure improvement for women. For example, some people erroneously advocate that trunk flexion from the standing position is an exercise to increase strength in the abdominal musculature. Trunk flexion from the standing position is *not* an exercise designed to develop abdominal muscle strength. People who indicate that it is have overlooked the effect of gravity on the organism.

Trunk flexion from the standing position is beneficial as a strengthening and flexibility exercise for the erector spinae both in spinal flexion and extension. The deep back muscles and erector spinae are the muscles most involved in lumbar flexion from the anatomic position because they are contracting eccentrically and actually control the degree of flexion. The abdominals, the contralateral muscles in this case, are relatively inactive owing to the fact that the head and trunk are being moved downward by the pull of gravity. The erector spinae are also the muscles most involved when the trunk is moved into extension against gravity from the flexed position. When the trunk is extended, the erector spinae must contract concentrically to overcome resistances provided by the head and trunk as well as gravity.

If the development of abdominal strength is the desired outcome of a given exercise, the body should be placed in a position so the pull of gravity serves as a resistance to be overcome. The most common position for this is the so-called "hook-lying position." The individual is in a supine position with the knees and hips flexed. The soles of the feet are kept flat on the floor, and the heels are approximately six inches from the buttocks. Trunk flexion performed from that position will develop abdominal strength because the abdominal musculature is the muscle group most involved for the movement against gravity. The five abdominal muscles most involved must contract concentrically to flex the trunk and overcome gravitational pull as well as the weight of the trunk and head. On the return to the floor or mat the abdominals continue to be the muscles most involved by contracting eccentrically and controlling the movement as the trunk and head are lowered slowly. It must be remembered that extension of the spine in this example is being done with gravity. The contractions of these muscle groups during the exercises described can be palpated.

The functions of the contralateral muscles often vary depending upon the skills being performed. Two major functions are (1) control of the speed of motion within the muscles most involved and (2) protection of the joint.

Guiding muscles are found on either side of the muscles most involved. Muscles within muscle groups have several potential actions which they can perform. When a desired action through a given plane of motion is performed, the guiding muscles provide a balance of pull on either side of the plane of motion. Therefore, the muscles most involved are allowed to perform as directed volitionally by the central nervous system. This does not rule out the possibility that guiding muscles may also be directly involved in a portion of the volitional movement. As an example, any individual movement can be performed at the hip joint through several ranges of motion, but it is possible to move through one plane of motion at a time. This requires teamwork between and among various muscle groups. When hip flexion is desired through the anteroposterior range of motion, this exact movement would be impossible if there were not muscles other than the muscles most involved for hip flexion to guide the total action. The abductors and adductors of the hip work in a teamwork fashion with the hip flexors to rule out undesired or rotary actions which might occur at the hip joint during flexion.

All muscle groups have the potential of being *stabilizing muscles.* Stabilization is often conceived as complete and prolonged isometric contraction of muscles surrounding a body part or joint. This is not the case in most sport or movement activities. Stabilization must be regarded as a relative concept, because movement to a greater or lesser degree is always taking place within joints considered to be stabilized. Owing to this factor, a different approach to stabilization is introduced as moving or *dynamic stabilization.* This appears paradoxical since the terms "dynamic" and "stabilizer" have opposite meanings. This is one of many paradoxes seen in muscle functions. This one is called the *Lomac Paradox.*

A consideration of dynamic stabilization is essential in the understanding of the timing aspect of sequential movements. Dynamic stabilization occurs within stabilizing muscle groups during a sport skill in instantaneous and fleeting bursts of muscle contractions. There are three major functions of dynamic stabilization. These may occur independently of each other or in an interrelated fashion during the performance of sport skills. These functions are (1) to maintain the position of the body against gravity, other external forces, and internal force generated by muscle contractions; (2) to prevent trauma within joints due to elongation or compression of the joint structure; or (3) to provide a base from which the original force desired to perform a sport skill can be initiated and transferred from one body segment to another body part in the desired direction or sequence of the skill.

The time element of dynamic stabilization within a joint or a body part is highly variable depending upon the sport skill and/or the amount of force to be overcome. For example, dynamic stabilization may occur for a relatively long period of time within a weight lifter's trunk and lower limb musculature when he is attempting to move maximum weight vertically during the two-hand military press. On the other hand, dynamic stabilization occurs within microseconds in upper and lower limb joints of a sprinter during a 100-yard dash.

SELECTED REFERENCES

1. ADAMS, ADRIAN. "Effect of Exercise Upon Ligament Strength." *Research Quarterly* 37:163-167, May, 1966.
2. AYERS, A. JEAN. "Levels of Central Integration of Sensorimotor Function." Unpublished report. Los Angeles: University of Southern California, 1961.
3. BASMAJIAN, JOHN V. "Electromyography of Two-Joint Muscles." *Anatomical Record* 129:371-80, November, 1957.
4. ELFTMAN, H. "The Action of Muscles in the Body." *Biological Symposium* 3:191-210, 1941.
5. HUBBARD, ALFRED W. "Homokinetics: Muscular Function in Human Movement." *Science and Medicine of Exercise and Sports.* Edited by Warren R. Johnson. New York: Harper & Row, Publishers, 1960.
6. LEVINE, M. G., and KABAT, H. "Cocontraction and Reciprocal Innervation in Voluntary Movement in Man." *Science* 116:115-118, 1952.
7. MONOD, H., and SCHERRER, J. "The Work Capacity of a Synergic Muscular Group." *Ergonomics* 8:329-38, July, 1965.
8. RAZUMORA, L. L., and FRANK, G. M. "An X-Ray Study of the Structure of Muscle Using Different Methods of Fixation." *Biophysics* 6:15-19, 1961.
9. SHERRINGTON, CHARLES SIR. *Man on His Nature.* Garden City: Doubleday & Company, Inc., 1955.
10. TAYLOR, JAMES, ed. *Selected Writings of John Hughlings Jackson*, Vol. 1. London: Hodder & Stoughton, Ltd., 1931.
11. WALLIS, EARL, and LOGAN, GENE A. *Figure Improvement and Body Conditioning Through Exercise.* Englewood Cliffs: Prentice-Hall, Inc., 1964.

lower limbs and pelvic girdle

▶ **Introduction**

In this chapter, as well as Chapters 6 and 7, the method of presenting aggregate muscle actions is the same. The emphasis is placed on surface anatomy because this is what the physical educator observes in teaching-coaching situations. In the introductory anatomy course, muscles are studied individually on cadavers. This is the first step in learning functional myology. In the basic kinesiology course, however, the future physical educator needs to gain a thorough understanding of aggregate muscle action and the teamwork between and among muscle groups.

To help conceptualize aggregate muscle actions for subsequent kinesiologic analyses, each muscle group is shown under tension at the joint involved by use of a photographic illustration. Accompanying each photographic illustration is a drawing which places an emphasis on the muscle group under study. The purpose of the drawing is to name and accentuate the location of the surface, or superficial, muscles. A study of the photographic and drawn illustrations as well as the text will assist the reader in conceptualizing the spatial relationship of a muscle group to the joints. Furthermore, it must be noted that each student possesses the same illustrated musculature. Palpating, naming, and describing these muscles under tension are very useful learning techniques.

The terms "proximal attachment" and "distal attachment" are used instead of the terms "origin" and "insertion." It is an anatomic fact that muscles do have the potential of reversing their pull at either end. The stabilized attachment may or may not be what is traditionally called the origin. It may be the insertion end of the muscle.

The concept of a relatively stable origin and an instable insertion tends to be misleading. For example, during the pull-up there is seen a reversal of function within the biceps brachii and brachialis muscles at

73

the elbow. The forearm is relatively stable as the upper arm flexes toward the forearm during the upward phase of the pull-up. Here it can be seen that the origin, or proximal attachment, of the biceps brachii in particular is actually the moving end. The same phenomenon is occurring in regard to the brachialis muscle. In addition to the terms "proximal" and "distal," the following terms will be used to describe muscle locations on the head and trunk: "superior," "inferior," "medial," and "lateral."

To better conceptualize the spatial relationship of a muscle to a joint, the muscle's line of pull or direction of pull as it crosses a joint must be clearly understood. When several muscles work as a group to move a joint through a desired plane of motion, the individual muscles within the group may have their line of pull directly within the movement plane or slightly diagonal to it. Generally, the muscles diagonal to the plane of motion serve a dual function as the *muscles most involved* to perform the movement and as guiding muscles for the movement. For example, dorsiflexion of the ankle, or talocrural, joint is performed by a group of four muscles: tibialis anterior, extensor hallucis longus, extensor digitorum longus, and peroneus tertius. The reference point for the line of pull for all muscles with the exception of those which move the toes and fingers is the midline of the body (sagittal plane). The proximal to distal line of pull of the tibialis anterior muscle is from lateral to medial. The line of pull of the extensor digitorum longus is slightly medial to lateral. The peroneus tertius also has a line of pull which is from medial to lateral, but it is more exaggerated than the extensor digitorum longus. The combined line of pull of these four muscles forms a fan-shaped configuration, and the tendons of these muscles converge together as they cross the ankle joint anteriorly. It is this *anterior spatial relationship* to the joint by the tendons of these four muscles which causes them to be the muscles most involved for dorsiflexion. The spatial relationship of the tibialis anterior and the peroneus tertius diagonal to the anteroposterior range of motion also enables them to act as guiding muscles during dorsiflexion. This kinesiologic principle has a general application to the study of aggregate muscle actions.

► ## Movements and Extrinsic Muscles of the Ankle Joint (Talocrural Joint)

The extrinsic muscles of the foot are discussed, and the intrinsic muscles, the muscles located entirely within the foot, are excluded. The extrinsic muscles have their proximal attachments outside the foot within the lower limb. The distal attachments are within the foot itself.

The movements of the ankle joint are *dorsiflexion* and *plantar flexion*. A slight amount of rotation may be possible within the ankle joint, but it is relatively insignificant to total ankle movement. It must be remembered that eversion and inversion *do not* take place at the ankle joint. They take place within the transverse tarsal and subtalar joints.

The two major purposes of the foot are weight bearing and locomotion. When executing a kinesiologic analysis of a sport performance, these must be taken into consideration because of their interrelationship. Morton has indicated that body weight should be evenly distributed between the forward weight-bearing aspect of the foot and the heel. (Morton, 1935) For example, a 120-pound person would bear sixty pounds of weight on each foot. Thirty pounds of weight would be borne on the calcaneus of each foot and thirty pounds distributed on the metatarsal heads of each foot. The weight borne on the metatarsal heads is further subdivided as follows: the lateral four heads have five pounds each, and the remaining ten pounds are distributed under the head of the first metatarsal. Deviations from this normal weight-bearing position in the upright stance will cause changes in bone and muscle relationships. This will result in undesirable locomotion patterns. It is obvious that weight bearing in various sport skills varies widely. The ability to shift and bear weight properly is one characteristic of a highly skilled performer.

The ankle joint is a relatively stable joint owing to its bony arrangement and the support provided by surrounding muscles and ligaments. The so-called instability of the ankle, which results in many athletic injuries, actually occurs at the subtalar and transverse tarsal joints. The malleoli of the tibia and fibula fit firmly over the talus. A series of ligaments help to support the ankle joint on all sides. The most lateral ligament is the calcaneofibular, and the most medial ligament is the deltoid ligament. These are often referred to as the collateral ligaments of the ankle. The deltoid ligament in particular has great tensile strength. This is necessary because of its dual function of providing ligamentous support for the ankle and longitudinal arch. The deltoid ligament is so strong that it may pull the bony attachment loose from the tibia before it will tear. Other ligaments support the ankle anteriorly and posteriorly.

The muscles at the ankle joint, as in all major joints of the body, are the most important joint stabilizers. The ligaments help to stabilize joints, but their major function is to prevent further movement within the range of motion at the joint's extreme limit. Muscular support of the ankle is strongest posteriorly. The lateral and medial muscular support is relatively weaker than the anterior muscular support.

The muscles most involved (MMI) in producing dorsiflexion against resistance are tibialis anterior, extensor hallucis longus, extensor digitorum longus, and peroneus tertius. The lines of pull of these muscles both individually and as a group were discussed in the example above. Their general spatial relationship to the talocrural joint is anterior (Figures 5.1 and 5.2).

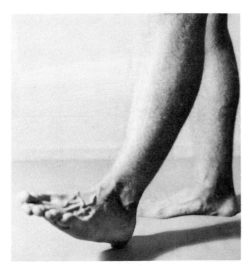

Figure 5.1. Dorsiflexion.

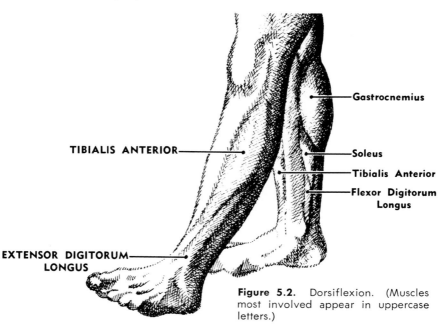

Gastrocnemius

TIBIALIS ANTERIOR

Soleus

Tibialis Anterior

Flexor Digitorum Longus

EXTENSOR DIGITORUM LONGUS

Figure 5.2. Dorsiflexion. (Muscles most involved appear in uppercase letters.)

Plantar flexion against resistance is performed by a group of seven muscles (MMI): gastrocnemius, soleus, peroneus longus, peroneus brevis, flexor digitorum longus, flexor hallucis longus, and tibialis posterior. The spatial relationship of the plantar flexor group to the ankle joint is posterior (Figures 5.3 and 5.4). The line of pull for the gastrocnemius

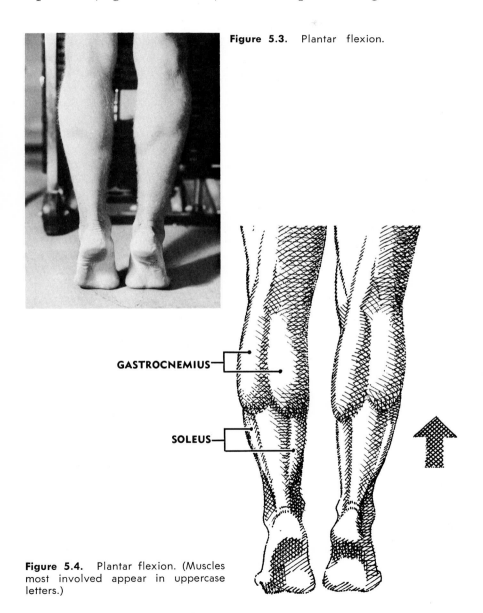

Figure 5.3. Plantar flexion.

GASTROCNEMIUS—

SOLEUS—

Figure 5.4. Plantar flexion. (Muscles most involved appear in uppercase letters.)

and soleus muscles is directly in the anteroposterior plane of motion. The peroneal muscles exert their force on the lateral aspect of the joint. Conversely, the flexor digitorum longus, flexor hallucis longus, and tibialis posterior serve as plantar flexors as well as guiding the action on the medial side of the ankle joint.

All guiding muscles for plantar flexion through the anteroposterior range of motion at the ankle joint work in a pulley fashion. On the lateral side, the peroneus longus and peroneus brevis utilize the lateral malleolus of the fibula as a pulley. Their tendons ride in a groove immediately posterior to the lateral malleolus as they move downward toward their distal attachments. On the medial side of the ankle, two guiding muscles—the flexor digitorum longus and tibialis posterior— function in a similar manner. Their tendons pass posterior to the medial malleolus via grooves enroute to their distal attachments. The tendon of the third medial guiding muscle for plantar flexion, the flexor hallucis longus, rides under the sustentaculum tali from the medial side of the calcaneus enroute to its distal attachment on the distal end of the great toe. The sustentaculum tali, like the medial and lateral malleoli, serve as a pulley for the flexor hallucis longus tendon. A critical observation of the spatial relationship and lines of pull of the guiding muscles for dorsiflexion and plantar flexion reveals that these muscles also function as inverters and everters of the subtalar and transverse tarsal joints. This is due to the fact that they are multiarticular muscles which cross those joints. Generally, if a muscle crosses a joint, it will act at that joint.

The term "triceps surae" is often used to describe the gastrocnemius and soleus muscles as one group. The prefix "tri" indicates that there are three basic structures to be considered. Confusion often exists regarding this point because there are only two muscles involved. The suffix "ceps" gives the answer to this problem. The term "ceps" means "heads." Thus, the term "triceps" refers to three muscle heads. In this case, there are three muscle heads in the two muscles. The gastrocnemius has two heads which attach proximally on the posterior aspects of the femoral condyles. The proximal head of the soleus attaches on the upper and posterior aspects of the tibia and fibula. The distal attachment for the triceps surae group is on the posterior surface of the calcaneus via the Achilles tendon. There is one other muscle which is sometimes missing in this area of the lower limb. It is called the plantaris. When present, the plantaris has its proximal attachment on the lateral aspect of the linea aspera of the femur and its distal attachment is via a long tendon to the posterior and medial aspect of the calcaneus. Since the plantaris is vestigial in man, it will not be discussed further.

Inversion takes place at the subtalar and transverse tarsal joints. The subtalar joint involves the articulation between the talus and calcaneus bones from below. The transverse tarsal joint involves articulations between the talus and navicular bones as well as the articulation between the calcaneus and cuboid bones. A group of five muscles work together as the muscles most involved (MMI) producing inversion: tibialis anterior, tibialis posterior, extensor hallucis longus, flexor hallucis longus, and flexor digitorum longus. The spatial relationship of these five muscles to the subtalar and transverse tarsal joints is medial (Figures 5.5 and 5.6).

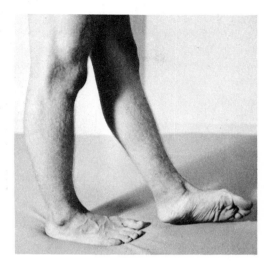

Figure 5.5. Inversion.

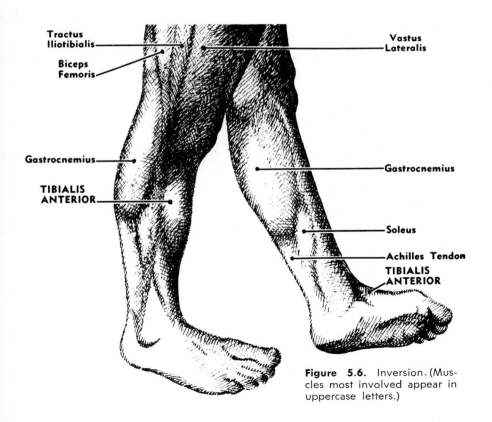

Tractus
Iliotibialis

Biceps
Femoris

Vastus
Lateralis

Gastrocnemius

**TIBIALIS
ANTERIOR**

Gastrocnemius

Soleus

Achilles Tendon

**TIBIALIS
ANTERIOR**

Figure 5.6. Inversion. (Muscles most involved appear in uppercase letters.)

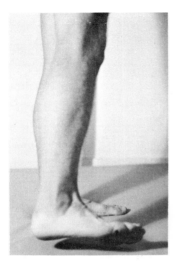

Figure 5.7. Eversion.

The guiding action is done during inversion by the three muscles which pass behind the medial malleolus. These are the tibialis posterior, flexor hallucis longus, and flexor digitorum longus. These muscles are also posterior to the plane of motion. The anterior set of guiding muscles during inversion consists of the extensor hallucis longus and tibialis anterior, i. e., they lie anterior to the plane of motion. When inversion occurs against resistance, these five muscles work as a group as the muscles most involved in performing the action, and they also guide the action through the lateral plane of motion simultaneously.

Eversion against resistance is done by a group of four muscles (MMI): ex-

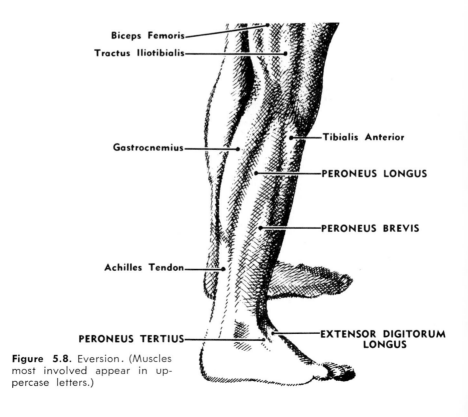

Biceps Femoris

Tractus Iliotibialis

Gastrocnemius

Tibialis Anterior

PERONEUS LONGUS

PERONEUS BREVIS

Achilles Tendon

PERONEUS TERTIUS

EXTENSOR DIGITORUM LONGUS

Figure 5.8. Eversion. (Muscles most involved appear in uppercase letters.)

tensor digitorum longus, peroneus tertius, peroneus longus, and peroneus brevis. The spatial relationship of these muscles to the subtalar and transverse tarsal joints is lateral (Figures 5.7 and 5.8).
These four muscles, while acting as the muscles most involved in producing eversion against resistance, also act as the guiding muscles for
the desired amount of eversion. The extensor digitorum longus and
peroneus tertius tendons are anterior to the lateral malleolus, and the
peroneus longus and peroneus brevis tendons "ride" posterior to the
lateral malleolus and have their distal attachments anterior and inferior
to it; consequently, the force exerted by these two pairs of muscles
against resistance tends to guide the foot as the four muscles combined
move it into an everted position against resistance.

Four extrinsic muscles of the foot are involved in flexion and extension at the metatarsophalangeal joints and interphalangeal joints. The
flexors are flexor digitorum longus and flexor hallucis longus. The extensors are extensor digitorum longus and extensor hallucis longus. These
muscles work in a teamwork fashion with the intrinsic muscles of the
foot to perform flexion and extension. The muscles which abduct and
adduct the toes are located entirely within the foot, i. e., they are intrinsic muscles of the foot.

▶ Movements of the Knee Joint

The movements possible at the knee joint are flexion, extension, medial
rotation, and lateral rotation. The rotary action possible in the knee is
only seen after flexion has occurred. Rotary movements are not observed
at the normal knee joint when it is fully extended. If there seems to be
rotation of the extended knee, a close examination will probably reveal
that rotation is occurring at the hip joint.

The knee is constructed to move most efficiently through the anteroposterior plane of motion. When the knees are used in such activities
as walking, jogging, sprinting, and running straight or on smooth surfaces, there are a limited number of potential hazards to damage the
knee. There are many times, however, when the knee undergoes extreme
stresses owing to the medial and lateral pivoting requirements of sport.
The knee must function effectively under the extreme stress of sport
competition to provide both mobility and stability for the performer.
Injuries often occur when the knee is placed in unnatural positions during
sport competition. Consequently, the supporting structures of the knee
should always be well conditioned to reduce the probability of injury.

Ligamentous support of the knee is relatively good; however, it
must be remembered that the major stability of the knee joint is derived
from muscle groups acting upon it. Relatively little stability is provided

by the bony articulation between the femoral condyles and the superior surface of the tibia. Bony stability is enhanced by the position of the medial and lateral menisci on the superior surface of the tibia. The menisci in this case tend to deepen the articulation.

There are two major pairs of ligaments which add anteroposterior and medial-lateral stability to the knee. These are the medial and lateral collateral ligaments which add stability in the lateral plane. The anterior and posterior cruciate ligaments add anteroposterior stability. The medial collateral ligament attaches the femur to the tibia. It also is attached to the medial meniscus. The lateral collateral ligament attaches the femur to the fibula but does not attach to the lateral meniscus. Both collateral ligaments lie slightly posterior to the lateral axis of the knee joint; therefore, they become taut when the knee is moved into complete extension. Conversely, the medial and lateral collateral ligaments become slack when the knee is flexed. This slackness of the collateral ligaments allows the knee to be rotated medially or laterally when the knee is flexed.

The cruciate ligaments are named because of their position of attachment on the superior head of the tibia. The term "cruciate" (*crux,* "to cross") implies that these two ligaments cross anteriorly and posteriorly within the septum of the knee joint. The anterior cruciate attaches to the tibia on its anterior-superior surface. It crosses through the knee joint from the medial side diagonally to its lateral attachment on the femur. The posterior cruciate attaches on the posterior-superior aspect of the tibia. It crosses diagonally and medially to its attachment on the femur. The cross-configuration of the cruciates adds stability to the knee joint when it is extended. In addition, the anterior cruciate prevents anterior movement of the tibia when the knee is flexed, and the posterior cruciate prevents posterior movement of the tibia while the knee is flexed. Other ligaments, including the capsular ligaments, provide additional stability for the knee joint.

The patellar ligament is misnamed. The patella is a sesamoid bone, i. e., it is a bone located within the quadriceps femoris tendon. Its posterior aspect articulates with the femur during flexion and extension at the knee joint. The structure usually identified as the patellar ligament is actually a continuation of the quadriceps femoris tendon attaching to the tibial tuberosity. Early anatomists assumed that the patellar ligament was actually attached to the patella and connected that bone with the tibia. Were this the case, it would meet the definition of a ligament because it would attach bone to bone. In effect, however, it attaches muscle to bone because of its continuation with the quadriceps femoris tendon.

The major stability for the knee joint comes from the muscles. The anterior stabilization of the knee joint is provided by the quadriceps femoris muscle group consisting of the rectus femoris, vastus medialis, vastus intermedius, and vastus lateralis. These four muscles converge into a common, fan-shaped tendon with its apex at the tibial tuberosity. This fan shape is important because it allows for more efficient use of the potential forces of the vastus medialis and vastus lateralis. Any other arrangement of the tendon would dissipate the internal forces generated by these muscles. It is rather interesting to observe that the middle fibers of the quadriceps femoris tendon are thicker than the lateral and medial fibers. The reason for this lies in the fact that this area of the tendon has tremendous forces exerted upon it by the rectus femoris *and* vastus intermedius muscles. Consequently, greater tensile strength of the tendon at this point is desired. These are the main muscles exerting force directly through the anteroposterior plane of motion for knee extension.

A high level of strength within the quadriceps femoris muscle group is important in preventing knee injury; consequently, weight-training programs should include resistance exercises for knee extension and flexion. Upon the initiation of a weight-training program, rapid gains in strength can be expected within the quadriceps femoris muscle group because most individuals have a relatively low level of strength within this muscle group. The potential strength is great in relation to other muscles, however, owing to the fact that the bipedal stance requires relatively little effort by the quadriceps muscle group in activities of daily living. The quadrupedal position probably demanded a muscle group the size of the quadriceps for locomotor purposes. This factor is also pertinent in regard to the relatively large size and potential strength of the gluteus maximus. Like the quadriceps femoris muscle group, the gluteus maximus in man is also relatively inactive in the bipedal stance during locomotion.

Posterior stabilization of the knee joint is due to actions of the gastrocnemius, popliteus, semitendinosus, semimembranosus, and biceps femoris muscles. Although the hamstring muscles—the semitendinosus, semimembranosus, and biceps femoris—are attached to the medial and lateral sides of the joint, they must be considered posterior muscles. The distal attachments of the hamstrings lie posterior to the axis of the joint. The hamstring muscles supply lateral and medial support as well as posterior support when the knee is extended. The gastrocnemius, discussed above, is also a posterior stabilizing muscle for the knee joint. Its proximal attachments are on the posterior aspects of the femoral condyles. These posterior attachments add to the stability of the knee when it is in extension. A companion muscle which functions with the gastrocnemius is the popliteus. The primary stability function for the popliteus is to prevent hyperextension of the knee.

Most of the lateral stability of the knee is derived secondarily from forces exerted by anterior and posterior muscle groups. Therefore, much stress and strain is placed on the medial and lateral collateral ligaments. This is one reason these ligaments are often injured in sport activities. Some lateral stability of the knee is given by the tractus iliotibialis, actually a lateral expansion or thickening of the fascia covering the entire thigh. It is thickened laterally to withstand the force exerted upon it at the level of the hip joint by the tensor fasciae latae and gluteus maximus muscles. In a rather remote fashion, the gluteus maximus and tensor fasciae latae add to the lateral stability of the knee also. At the same time, they maintain tension on the fascia surrounding the musculature of the total thigh. On the medial side of the knee, the gracilis and sartorius are in a position to maintain minimal stability of the knee joint when it is extended.

The four muscles most involved for knee extension against resistance are within the quadriceps femoris muscle group: rectus femoris, vastus medialis, vastus intermedius, and vastus lateralis. These four muscles have an anterior spatial relationship to the knee joint (Figures 5.9 and 5.10). In general, the three vasti muscles envelope the femur. The vastus medialis and vastus lateralis are the only two vasti muscles which can be palpated. The vastus intermedius lies between the vastus medialis and vastus lateralis; however, the rectus femoris is superficial to the vastus intermedius. It is the rectus femoris muscle lying between the vastus lateralis and vastus medialis which is palpable on the anterior aspect of the thigh. The vasti muscles are uniarticular with their function at the knee joint only. The rectus femoris is a biarticular muscle with movement functions at knee and hip joints.

The lines of pull of the rectus femoris and vastus intermedius muscles are directly within the anteroposterior plane of motion for knee extension. The line of pull of the vastus lateralis is from lateral to medial, and the line of pull of the vastus medialis is from medial to lateral. As a result, they serve a dual role as the muscles most involved for knee extension as well as a minimal guiding function during knee extension. The major guiding muscles during knee extension, however, are the hamstring muscles. In this instance the contralateral muscles also serve as guiding muscles.

Knee flexion against resistance is performed by a group of seven muscles. Of these, three have a distinct mechanical advantage for knee flexion. Consequently, they are the muscles most involved in this action. These MMI are the semitendinosus, semimembranosus, and biceps femoris muscles. The four remaining knee flexors are the sartorius, gracilis, popliteus, and gastrocnemius. The latter four muscles serve a secondary function during knee flexion against resistance. The seven muscles most

Figure 5.9. Knee extension.

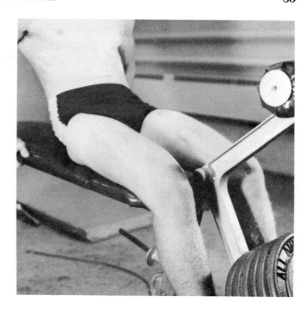

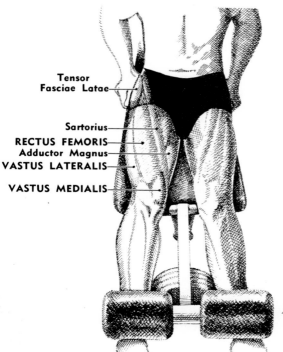

Figure 5.10. Knee extension. (Muscles most involved appear in uppercase letters.)

Tensor
Fasciae Latae

Sartorius

RECTUS FEMORIS
Adductor Magnus
VASTUS LATERALIS

VASTUS MEDIALIS

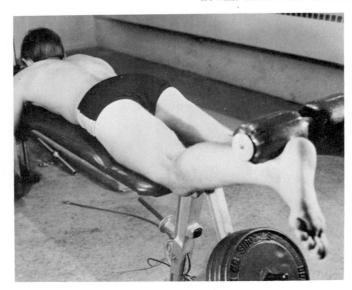

Figure 5.11.   Knee flexion.

involved for knee flexion are contralateral to the four muscles involved in knee extension. The spatial relationship of the popliteus and gastrocnemius muscles is directly posterior to the knee joint. The semitendinosus, semimembranosus, sartorius, and gracilis have their distal attachments medial to the joint, and the biceps femoris muscle has its distal attachment lateral to the joint. However, all five of these muscles have their distal attachments posterior to the lateral axis of the knee joint. This posterior spatial relationship to the knee joint makes them knee flexors (Figures 5.11 and 5.12).

Rotation of the knee joint is only possible when the knee is flexed. Medial rotation of the knee against resistance is done by a group of five muscles (MMI): semitendinosus, semimembranosus, popliteus, sartorius, and gracilis. These five muscles have their distal attachments on the medial aspect of the tibial condyle. Consequently, when the knee is moved into flexion, their pull during concentric contraction moves the knee into medial rotation unless the force is counteracted by the contralateral muscle, the biceps femoris.

The biceps femoris has its distal attachment on the head of the fibula and lateral condyle of the tibia; as a result, when it contracts concentrically against resistance while the knee is being flexed, it is the muscle most involved to rotate the knee laterally unless its force is counteracted by the five medial rotators of the knee. The muscles which

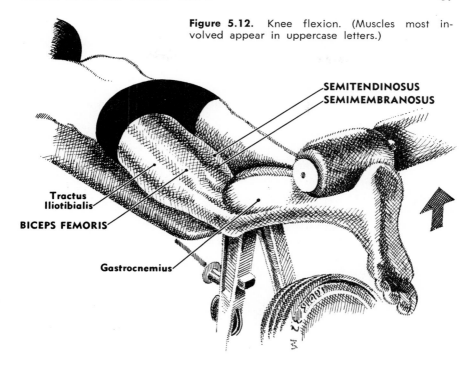

Figure 5.12. Knee flexion. (Muscles most involved appear in uppercase letters.)

SEMITENDINOSUS
SEMIMEMBRANOSUS

Tractus
Iliotibialis

BICEPS FEMORIS

Gastrocnemius

perform medial and lateral rotation also serve as guiding muscles for knee extension through the anteroposterior range of motion.

▶ Movements of the Hip, or Coxal, Joint

Movements possible at the hip joint include flexion, extension, adduction, abduction, diagonal abduction, diagonal adduction, medial and lateral rotation, and circumduction. Although the hip joint is supported anteriorly by a large amount of connective tissue, posteriorly there is a wide range and variety of movement within this joint. The hip joint is a very stable structure because of its bone and ligamentous arrangement as well as its muscular support.

The bony stability results from the relationship between the deep, cuplike acetabulum of the pelvis and the head of the femur. The femoral head is actually received within the acetabulum area. This type of bony articulation is needed because the hip joint must bear considerable weight in the bipedal stance.

Ligamentous support is mainly anterior to the hip joint. Primarily responsible for hip joint stability is the iliofemoral ligament. This ligament is commonly called the "Y" ligament. The pubofemoral ligament provides additional support. The iliofemoral ligament is one of the strongest ligaments in the body and limits extension of the hip. There is no analogous structure for preventing hip flexion. One other ligamentous structure which provides a limited amount of stability at the hip joint is the teres ligament. This ligament connects the head of the femur to the concave surface of the acetabulum.

Although there is considerable bony and ligamentous support to maintain stability of the hip joint, the major stabilizing force is provided by the muscles surrounding the hip joint. Posterior stabilization of the hip joint comes from the semitendinosus, semimembranosus, biceps femoris, and gluteus maximus. Anterior stabilization, from a muscular standpoint, is provided mainly by the iliopsoas and rectus femoris muscles. However, the iliofemoral ligament provides a great amount of anterior stabilization with the hip extended. Lateral stabilization is due primarily to the interaction of the gluteus minimus, gluteus medius, and tensor fasciae latae muscles, with some help from the gluteus maximus. The muscles have a tendency to counteract the gravitational pull downward. There is an analogy between the actions of these four muscles and the three parts of the deltoid muscle at the shoulder joint. Without these muscles the pelvis would tend to drop on the opposite side during unilateral weight bearing.

The lateral stabilizers are called upon to act at their highest level in a unilateral weight-bearing position. The relationship between the femur and the pelvis is architecturally a cantilever construction. The concentric contraction of the gluteus medius in the unilateral weight-bearing position has a tendency to draw the crest of the ilium down toward the femur on the same side which, in turn, causes lateral pelvic girdle rotation on the opposite side. This is a basic concept which must be understood in virtually all sport skills. For example, this action is seen during running. When the foot strikes the ground and becomes the weight-bearing limb, the lateral stabilizers of the hip on that side must hold the pelvis in position so the opposite limb, the non-weight-bearing limb, can go through the so-called "free-swinging" phase of running. During this "free-swinging" phase, all body weight is borne by the hip joint on the weight-bearing side. At this time, the major function of unilateral weight bearing is assumed by the gluteus minimus, gluteus medius, tensor fasciae latae, and gluteus maximus muscles. Analyses of running and sprinting performances by athletes should be thought of as a sequential and alternating series of unilateral weight-bearing movements.

Medial stabilization of the hip joint by muscles is the direct result of the adductor muscle group: the adductor longus, adductor brevis, and adductor magnus muscles. These muscles are assisted in this stabilization function by the gracilis and pectineus muscles.

The muscles most involved in hip joint flexion against resistance are the psoas, iliacus, rectus femoris, tensor fasciae latae, and pectineus (Figures 5.13 and 5.14). At the hip joint, the iliacus and psoas can be

Figure 5.13. Hip flexion.

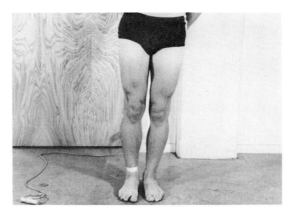

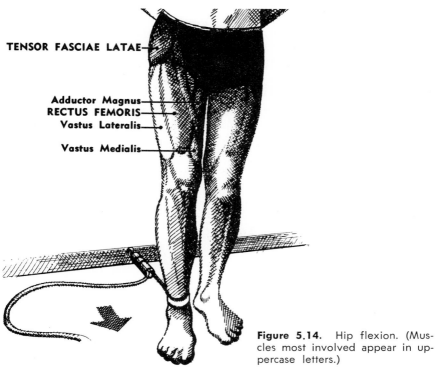

TENSOR FASCIAE LATAE

Adductor Magnus
RECTUS FEMORIS
Vastus Lateralis

Vastus Medialis

Figure 5.14. Hip flexion. (Muscles most involved appear in uppercase letters.)

thought of as one muscle, the iliopsoas. These five hip joint flexors all have an *anterior* spatial relationship to the joint which enhances their leverage potential. Several other muscles are also involved in the action of hip flexion. The medial guiding muscles for hip flexion are the sartorius, gracilis, adductor longus, adductor brevis, and upper fibers of the adductor magnus. Laterally, the guiding muscles are the tensor fasciae latae, gluteus minimus, and gluteus medius. As stated previously, guiding muscles can function as muscles most involved as well as guiders. The contralateral muscles for hip flexion are the muscles posterior to the hip joint—the hip extensors.

The muscles most involved in hip joint extension against resistance are the gluteus maximus, long head of the biceps femoris, semitendinosus, and semimembranosus. Their spatial relationship to the hip joint is posterior (Figures 5.15 and 5.16). Medial guiding muscles for hip joint extension are the adductor brevis, adductor longus, adductor magnus, and gracilis. The lateral guiding muscles for hip joint extension are the gluteus medius, piriformis, obturator internus, obturator externus, quadratus femoris, gemellus superior, and gemellus inferior. The latter six muscles are commonly grouped together functionally, because they are all small lateral rotators of the hip joint.

The muscle most involved in hip abduction is the gluteus medius. This muscle has a direct lateral spatial relationship to the hip joint (Figures 5.17 and 5.18). The anterior guiding muscles for abduction of the hip are the iliopsoas, sartorius, rectus femoris, tensor fasciae latae, and gluteus minimus. Posteriorly, the guiding muscles for hip abduction are the gluteus maximus, long head of the biceps femoris, semitendinosus, semimembranosus, and the six small lateral rotators of the hip referred to above.

Hip adduction against resistance is performed by the adductor brevis, adductor longus, adductor magnus, and gracilis. These muscles have a medial spatial relationship to the hip joint (Figures 5.19 and 5.20). The guiding muscles for hip adduction on the anterior side are the pectineus, iliopsoas, sartorius, rectus femoris, and tensor fasciae latae. The posterior guiding muscles for hip adduction are the gluteus maximus, long head of the biceps femoris, semitendinosus, and semimembranosus.

Diagonal adduction is a movement at the hip joint through the diagonal plane of motion for the lower limb. Diagonal adduction, as seen in sport, consists of a combination of three traditional movements: (1) adduction, (2) flexion, and (3) medial rotation. The muscles involved in diagonal adduction are in a much more favorable position for the performance of this movement as opposed to straight adduction or hip flexion.

Figure 5.15. Hip extension.

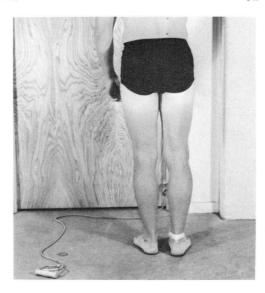

Figure 5.16. Hip extension. (Muscles most involved appear in uppercase letters.)

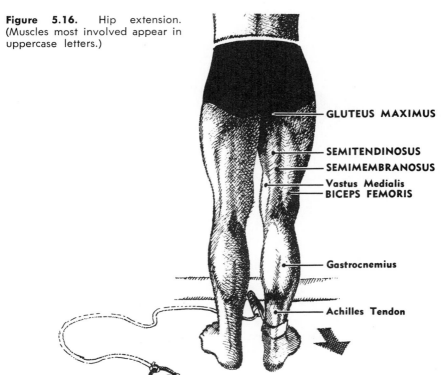

GLUTEUS MAXIMUS

SEMITENDINOSUS

SEMIMEMBRANOSUS

Vastus Medialis
BICEPS FEMORIS

Gastrocnemius

Achilles Tendon

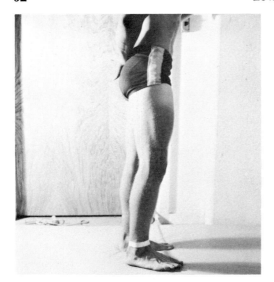

Figure 5.17. Hip abduction.

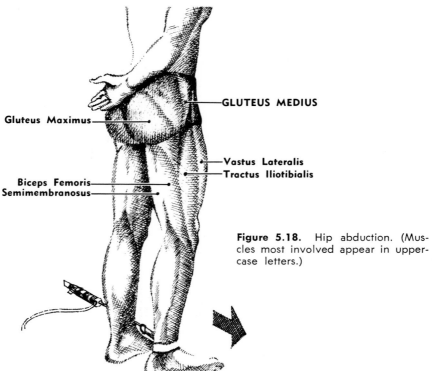

GLUTEUS MEDIUS

Gluteus Maximus

Vastus Lateralis
Tractus Iliotibialis

Biceps Femoris
Semimembranosus

Figure 5.18. Hip abduction. (Muscles most involved appear in uppercase letters.)

Figure 5.19. Hip adduction.

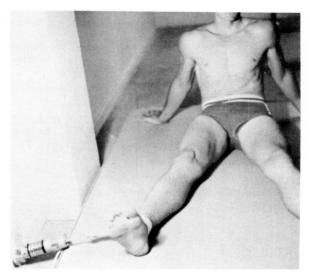

Figure 5.20. Hip adduction. (Muscles most involved appear in uppercase letters.)

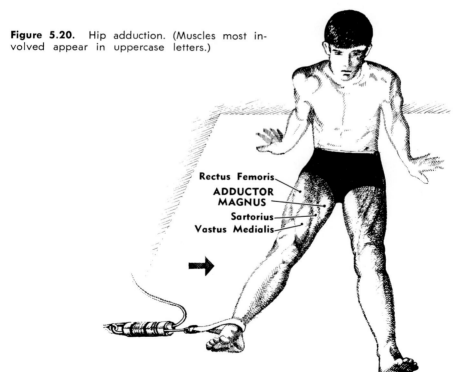

Rectus Femoris
ADDUCTOR MAGNUS
Sartorius
Vastus Medialis

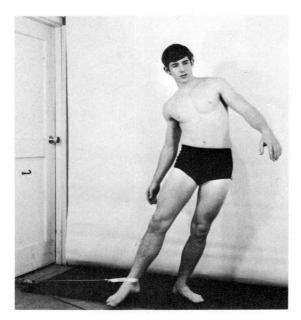

Figure 5.21. Hip diagonal adduction.

One way that hip joint diagonal adduction is used in sport is by
the soccer player who kicks the ball with the medial aspect of the foot.
At the beginning of the soccer-style kick, the hip joint is abducted,
laterally rotated, and extended to place the muscles most involved for
diagonal adduction on their longest length. These three movements
combined constitute diagonal abduction. The kicker starts diagonal adduction from this position. As a consequence, he calls upon the adductors,
hip flexors, and medial rotators of the hip.

In terms of muscle mass involvement, more potential internal force
is available for diagonal adduction than in any single action of the three
traditional movements. Consequently, this is one reason why relatively
small soccer-style kickers obtain great distances in their kicks. This is
also one reason that this style of kicking is being adopted by American
football place-kickers. These larger men will be able to get great distances using diagonal adduction once they have mastered the kicking
skill. It will be remembered that most American football place-kickers
use a toe-kicking style employing hip flexion and knee extension through
the anteroposterior plane of motion. In American-style place-kicking a
relatively small amount of the foot surface contacts the ball; whereas,
in soccer-style kicking a large portion of the medial aspect of the foot
comes into contact with the football. This has a tendency to result in
greater accuracy as well as distance.

Figure 5.22. Hip diagonal adduction. (Muscles most involved appear in uppercase letters.)

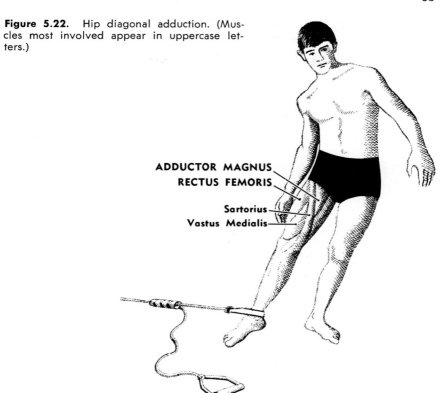

ADDUCTOR MAGNUS
RECTUS FEMORIS
Sartorius
Vastus Medialis

The muscles most involved for diagonal adduction against resistance are the iliopsoas, rectus femoris, pectineus, adductor magnus, adductor longus, and adductor brevis (Figures 5.21 and 5.22). The medial guiding muscle for diagonal adduction is provided by the gracilis. The lateral guiding muscles are the tensor fasciae latae, gluteus minimus, and gluteus medius. The contralateral muscles for diagonal adduction are the gluteus maximus, semitendinosus, semimembranosus, long head of the biceps femoris, and the six lateral rotators. These muscles become the muscles most involved for diagonal abduction against resistance (Figures 5.23 and 5.24).

The muscles most involved in medial rotation of the hip against resistance are the tensor fasciae latae, gluteus minimus, and anterior fibers of the gluteus medius (Figures 5.25 and 5.26). The muscles most involved for lateral rotation against resistance are the gluteus maximus, posterior fibers of the gluteus medius, and the six lateral rotators of the hip (Figures 5.27 and 5.28).

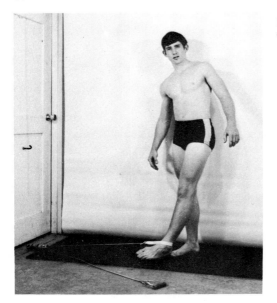

Figure 5.23. Hip diagonal abduction.

Figure 5.24. Hip diagonal abduction. (Muscles most involved are not seen in anterior view.)

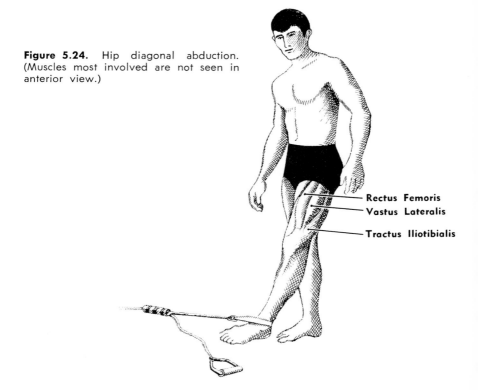

Rectus Femoris

Vastus Lateralis

Tractus Iliotibialis

Figure 5.25. Hip medial rotation.

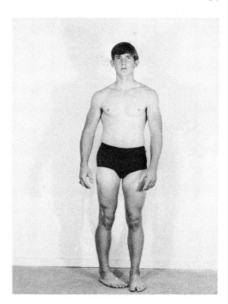

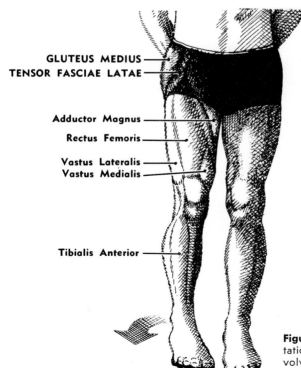

GLUTEUS MEDIUS
TENSOR FASCIAE LATAE

Adductor Magnus
Rectus Femoris

Vastus Lateralis
Vastus Medialis

Tibialis Anterior

Figure 5.26. Hip medial rotation. (Muscles most involved appear in uppercase letters.)

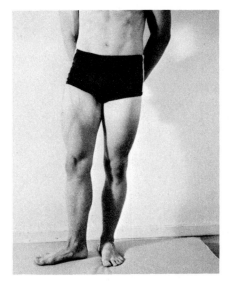

Figure 5.27. Hip lateral rotation.

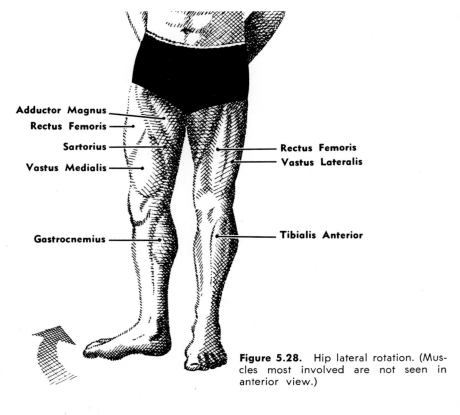

Adductor Magnus

Rectus Femoris

Sartorius

Vastus Medialis

Rectus Femoris

Vastus Lateralis

Gastrocnemius

Tibialis Anterior

Figure 5.28. Hip lateral rotation. (Muscles most involved are not seen in anterior view.)

▶ The Pelvic Girdle

New terminology for pelvic girdle movements was introduced in Chapter 2. The discussion at this point concerns aggregate muscle actions for pelvic girdle movements while the individual is in a (1) standing position with the weight distributed on the feet or on one foot and (2) hanging position with the weight borne by the hands. These movements are used in conjunction with other movements taking place in a sequential fashion during sport, exercise, and dance. There are many times in sport, for example, when there is a transfer of internal forces occurring through the pelvic girdle to the trunk or from the pelvic girdle to the lower limb. From a noncinematographic analysis standpoint, the observer can "key" on pelvic girdle movements to observe such things as weight shift, transfer of forces, line of thrust for the center of mass, and other pertinent factors of motion.

There is often a reversal of function by muscles connected to the pelvic girdle. As an example, while the muscles of the upper trunk are stabilizing the rib cage, the muscles attached to the pelvis from above are capable of moving the pelvic girdle. On the other hand, while the lower limbs are stabilized, the musculature attached to the pelvis from below will move the pelvic girdle.

Movements by the *pelvic girdle* are as follows: right transverse pelvic rotation, left transverse pelvic rotation, anterior pelvic rotation, posterior pelvic rotation, right lateral pelvic rotation, and left lateral pelvic rotation.

The muscles most involved in right transverse pelvic rotation against resistance when the athlete is in a *hanging position* are the right external oblique muscle and the left internal oblique muscle. The pelvis in this case is rotated to the individual's right. The contralateral muscles for right transverse pelvic rotation are the left external oblique and the right internal oblique. When the performer is bearing his weight on both feet, the muscles most involved for right transverse pelvic rotation are the right gluteus maximus and the left tensor fasciae latae, left gluteus minimus and anterior fibers of the left gluteus medius. The contralateral muscles for right transverse pelvic rotation are the left gluteus maximus and right tensor fasciae latae, right gluteus minimus and anterior fibers of the right gluteus medius. The contralateral muscles listed in the discussion of right transverse pelvic rotation are the muscles most involved for left transverse pelvic rotation. (Figure 5.29, p. 100)

Anterior pelvic rotation occurs when the iliac crests move forward through the anteroposterior plane of motion. When the performer is hanging by his hands, the muscles most involved in anterior pelvic rotation are located within the erector spinae muscle group. The contralateral

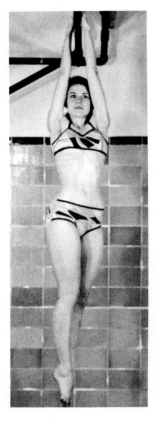

Figure 5.29. Left transverse pelvic girdle rotation.

muscle for anterior pelvic rotation is the rectus abdominis. When the individual is in a weight-bearing position, some caution must be given to ascribing muscle action to pelvic movements because the effect of gravity *and* resistance must be brought into consideration (Figure 5.30). For example, while doing a hip flexion exercise by pulling on a heavy wall-pulley device or an Exer-Genie Exerciser from above, the muscles most involved in anterior pelvic rotation, which accompanies hip flexion in this case, are the hip flexors. These are the rectus femoris, iliopsoas, and pectineus muscles. The contralateral muscles in anterior pelvic rotation against resistance are the gluteus maximus, semitendinosus, semimembranosus, and biceps femoris. While in the standing position, with the trunk being flexed slowly by the pull of gravity, there is concurrent hip flexion and anterior pelvic rotation. The muscles most involved in this anterior pelvic rotation are the gluteus maximus, semitendinosus, semimembranosus, and long head of the biceps femoris. These muscles are allowing rotation to occur in the pelvic girdle by contracting eccentrically. The muscles contralateral to anterior pelvic rotation in the weight-bearing position are the pectineus, rectus femoris, and iliopsoas.

The muscles most involved for posterior pelvic girdle rotation while standing on both feet are gluteus maximus, semitendinosus, semimembranosus, long head of the biceps femoris, six lateral rotators, and rectus abdominis (Figure 5.31).

Lateral pelvic girdle rotation occurs both right and left. When the individual is hanging by his hands, the muscles most involved in right lateral pelvic girdle rotation are the erector spinae on the right side and the three abdominal muscles on the right side excluding the transverse abdominis. The contralateral muscles in right lateral pelvic girdle rotation are the left erector spinae and the left side of the three abdominal muscles excluding the transverse abdominis. In a unilateral weight-bearing position with the weight being distributed through the individual's left leg, right lateral pelvic rotation is a result of concentric

Figure 5.30. Anterior pelvic girdle rotation.

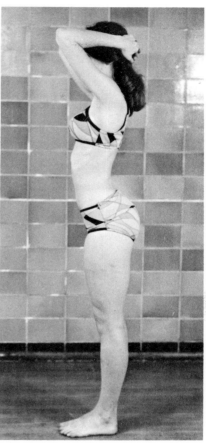

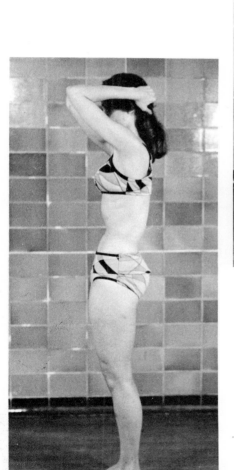

Figure 5.31. Posterior pelvic girdle rotation.

contraction by the left gluteus medius (Figure 5.32). The right gluteus medius is the muscle most involved for left lateral pelvic rotation. The contralateral muscles for this action are the adductor longus, adductor magnus, and adductor brevis on the left leg.

Side-to-side shifting movement of the pelvis is not to be confused with lateral pelvic girdle rotation. The side-to-side shifting movement of the pelvis in the lateral plane is simply a matter of adduction and abduction of the hip joint. The crest of the ilium remains relatively level when abduction and adduction are occurring within this context when weight is distributed over both feet.

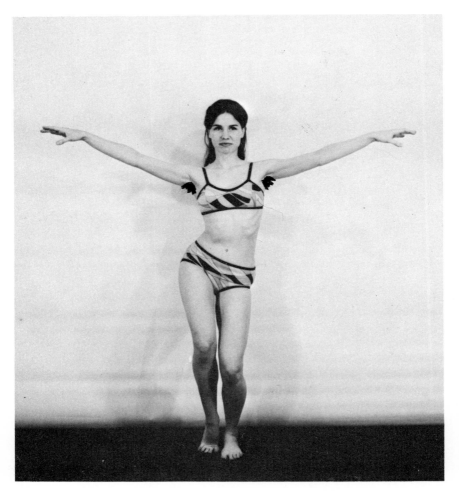

Figure 5.32. Right lateral pelvic girdle rotation.

SELECTED REFERENCES

1. ALLINGTON, RUTH OWNE, and OTHERS. "Strengthening Techniques of the Quadriceps Muscles: An Electromyographic Evaluation." *Physical Therapy* 46:1173-76, November, 1966.
2. BASMAJIAN, JOHN V., and STECKO, GEORGE. "The Role of Muscles in Arch Support of the Foot." *Journal of Bone and Joint Surgery* 45A:1184-90, September, 1963.
3. BIERMAN, WILLIAM, and RALSTON, H. J. "Electromyographic Study During Passive and Active Flexion and Extension of the Knee of the Normal Human Subject." *Archives of Physical Medicine and Rehabilitation* 46:71-75, January, 1965.
4. BREWERTON, D. A. "The Function of the Vastus Medialis Muscle." *Annals of Physical Medicine* 2:164-168, 1955.
5. CAVAGNA, G. A., and MARGARIA, R. "Mechanics of Walking." *Journal of Applied Physiology* 21:271-78, January, 1966.
6. DEMPSTER, W. T. "The Range of Motion of Cadaver Joints: The Lower Limb." *University of Michigan Medical Bulletin* 22:364-79, 1956.
7. ELFTMAN, H. "Forces and Energy Changes in the Leg During Walking." *American Journal of Physiology* 125:339-356, 1959.
8. GOLLNICK, PHILIP D. "Electrogoniometric Study of Walking on High Heels." *Research Quarterly* 35:370-78, October, 1964.
9. GRIEVE, D. W., and GEAR, RUTH J. "The Relationships Between Length of Stride, Step Frequence, Time of Swing and Speed of Walking for Children and Adults." *Ergonomics* 9:379-99, September, 1966.
10. HALL, W. L., and KLEIN, K. K. "The Man, the Knee and the Ligaments." *Medicina Dello Sport* 1:50Q-11, October, 1961.
11. HALLEN, L. G., and LINDAHL, O. "The Lateral Stability of the Knee Joint." *Acta Orthopaedica Scandinavica* 36:179-191, 1965.
12. ———. "The 'Screw-Home' Movement in the Knee Joint." *Acta Orthopaedica Scandinavica* 37:97-106, Fasc. 1, 1966.
13. HOUTZ, S. J., and WALSH, FRANK P. "Electromyographic Analysis of the Function of the Muscles Acting on the Ankle During Weight Bearing with Special Reference to the Triceps Surae." *Journal of Bone and Joint Surgery* 41-A:1469-1481, 1959.
14. INMAN, VERNE T. "Functional Aspects of the Abductor Muscles of the Hip." *Journal of Bone and Joint Surgery* 29:607-619, 1947.
15. JONSSON, BENGT, and STEEN, BERTIL. "Function of the Gracilis Muscle." *Acta Morphologica Neerlando-Scandinavica* 6:325-341, 1966.
16. KAPLAN, EMANUEL B. "The Iliotibial Tract." *Journal of Bone and Joint Surgery* 40-A:817-832, 1958.
17. KARPOVICH, PETE V., and WILKLOW, LEIGHTON B. "Goniometric Study of the Human Foot in Standing and Walking." *Industrial Medicine and Surgery* 29:338-347, July, 1960.
18. KLEIN, KARL K. "The Deep Squat Exercise as Utilized in Weight Training for Athletics and Its Effect on the Ligaments of the Knee." *Journal of the Association for Physical and Mental Rehabilitation* 15:6-11, January-February, 1961.
19. ———. "The Knee and the Ligaments." *Journal of Bone and Joint Surgery* 44-A:1191-1193, September, 1962.
20. LAWRENCE, MARY S., MEYER, HARRIET R., and MATTHEWS, NANCY L. "Comparative Increase in Music Strength in the Quadriceps Femoris by

Isometric and Isotonic Exercises and Effects on the Contralateral Muscle." *Journal of the American Physical Therapy Association* 42:15-20, January, 1962.

21. MATHEWS, DONALD, SHAW, VIRGINIA, and BOHNEN, MELRA. "Hip Flexibility of College Women as Related to Length of Body Segments." *Child Development Abstracts and Bibliography* 32:85, June-August, 1958.

22. MATHEWS, DONALD K., SHAW, VIRGINIA, and WOODS JOHN B. "Hip Flexibility of Elementary School Boys as Related to Body Segments." *Research Quarterly* 30:297-302, October, 1959.

23. MORTON, DUDLEY J. *The Human Foot.* New York: Columbia University Press, 1935.

24. O'CONNELL, A. L. "Electromyographic Study of Certain Leg Muscles During Movements of the Free Foot and During Standing." *American Journal of Physical Medicine* 37:289-301, December, 1958.

25. RARICK, L., and THOMPSON, J. "Roentgenographic Measures of Leg Muscle Size and Ankle Extensor Strength." *Research Quarterly* 27:321, October, 1956.

26. RICCI, BENJAMIN, and KARPOVICH, PETER V. "Effect of Height of Heel Upon the Foot." *Research Quarterly* 35:385-88, October, 1964.

27. SHEFFIELD, F. J., and OTHERS. "Electromyographic Study of the Muscles of the Foot in Normal Walking." *American Journal of Physical Medicine* 35:223-236, 1956.

28. SUTHERLAND, DAVID H. "An Electromyographic Study of the Plantar Flexors of the Ankle in Normal Walking on the Level." *Journal of Bone and Joint Surgery* 48-A:66-71, January, 1966.

29. WHEATLEY, M. D., and JOHNKE, W. D. "Electromyographic Study of the Superficial Thigh and Hip Muscles in Normal Individuals." *Archives of Physical Medicine* 32:508-515, 1951.

the spinal column and rib cage

The spinal column consists of seven vertebrae in the cervical, or neck, area, twelve in the thoracic area, and five in the lumbar area. Movement within and between these twenty-four vertebrae is extensive; however, movement between any two vertebrae is relatively small. The majority of motion occurs at the cervical and lumbar areas of the spine. The thoracic area, including the rib cage, is a relatively stable or fixed portion of the spinal column. In addition to the twenty-four vertebrae in the cervical, thoracic, and lumbar areas, five fixed vertebrae compose the sacrum, and four partially movable vertebrae comprise the coccyx. Thus, the spinal column consists of thirty-three vertebrae.

The twelve thoracic vertebrae and the rib cage to which they are attached can be considered as one functional unit. This unit has a limited degree of movement potential with the exception of rib movement required in breathing. From a kinesiologic standpoint, this unit can be thought of as a constant volumetric structure because the rib cage, unlike the lungs, does not change its size appreciably during gross movement.

Functioning with the thoracic spine-rib cage unit to make up what is commonly known as the "trunk" is the pelvic girdle. The pelvic girdle, like the thoracic rib cage area, can also be thought of as a functional unit. These two units of the trunk are joined together by the lumbar vertebrae. The lumbar vertebrae can be considered a pivotal support structure linking the two units together. With the exception of the psoas, the muscles connecting the pelvic girdle to the rib cage anterior, lateral, and posterior are the muscles which cause motion to occur within the lumbar spine.

The seven cervical vertebrae function as another pivotal support structure. These vertebrae serve as a connective link between the rib cage and the head. This area, the neck, is moved by muscles connecting

105

the rib cage to the head. The head, like the rib cage, can be thought of as a nonchanging volumetric structure. Thus it can be seen that in the so-called trunk area there are three nonchanging volumetric units connected by two pivotal support structures. As a result, virtually all movements of the spinal column take place within the two supportive areas known as the lumbar and cervical portions of the spine. For kinesiologic analysis purposes, it is suggested that the individual focus attention primarily on six separate segments of the body. These six important segments are (1) pelvic girdle, (2) rib cage, (3) head, (4) shoulder girdle, (5) upper limbs, and (6) lower limbs. Generally, when analyzing any sport skill the observer should start with a critical observation of the pelvic region of the performer.

All possible motions are seen within the various units of the spinal column and occur between the facets of the vertebrae which lie posterior to the longitudinal axis of the spinal column. Motions possible within the lumbar and cervical spinal column segments are flexion, extension, diagonal flexion, diagonal extension, rotation around the longitudinal axis, and lateral flexion.

In general, the entire spinal column has relatively good ligamentous support given to it by short, strong ligaments connecting individual vertebrae. The most important of these are the anterior longitudinal ligament, posterior longitudinal ligament, and the ligamentum nuchae. The anterior longitudinal ligament is continuous from the occipital bone to the sacrum. It is relatively thin in the cervical region and thick in the thoracic region. The posterior longitudinal ligament is continuous from the occipital bone to the coccygeal region. The ligamentum nuchae is located in the posterior cervical region. It is a continuation of the supraspinous ligament from the seventh cervical vertebra to the occipital region. It is a strong, but thin, fibrous membrane in this area. The supraspinous ligament is actually a continuation of the ligamentum nuchae from the seventh cervical vertebra to the sacrum. The supraspinous ligament and its continuation in the cervical region, the ligamentum nuchae, help to maintain the spinal column in an erect position. In this regard, they function as antigravity ligaments adding to the extension capacity of the antigravity musculature.

The bony support between the articulations of the spinal column is relatively unstable. The main bony support is posterior. The spinous processes, for example, serve as limiting structures for extension and hyperextension of the spine. There also is some bony support in the area of the rib cage. This is provided by the articulation of the ribs with the articular facets of the vertebrae in the thoracic area.

Muscle stability within the spinal area is of vital importance. The muscles connecting the pelvic girdle to the rib cage as well as the muscular connection of the rib cage to the head serve as dynamic stabilizers when required for movements of the upper and lower limbs. Because man has assumed the bipedal, or upright, position, the muscles in the lumbar region are required to do less work than they would in a flexed, or quadrupedal, position. Consequently, the strength of these muscles is usually much less than their potential strength level. In addition, the muscles connecting the pelvic girdle to the rib cage are often overlooked in the conditioning process for sport skills involving the use of the limbs. In terms of maximum performance in sports, these two factors must be considered, especially during the training or conditioning process.

▶ Lumbar Spine Movements

Movements of the lumbar spine are discussed in terms of the most important muscles only. These are the rectus abdominis, external oblique, internal oblique, and the erector spinae group collectively. From a kinesiologic standpoint, these muscles must be considered when the individual is in weight-bearing and non-weight-bearing positions. This is necessary to conceptualize the relationship between the reversal of muscle function and dynamic stabilization.

The muscles most involved in lumbar flexion against resistance are the rectus abdominis, external oblique, and internal oblique muscles. These muscles have an anterior spatial relationship to the lumbar vertebrae. When the individual is in a supine position with his hips and knees flexed and feet flat on the floor (hook-lying position), movement of the rib cage toward the thighs is done by these muscles. The line of pull of the rectus abdominis in this example is directly in the anteroposterior plane of motion. The external and internal oblique muscles are among the muscles most involved in this movement, but they are also guiding muscles for this action. (Abdominal musculature is seen in Figures 6.1 and 6.2.) The principal reason for this is that the internal and external obliques also have the capacity to rotate the lumbar spine. However, when pulling equally and bilaterally they perform flexion and counteract their rotary actions. The contralateral muscles for this action consist of the muscles found in the erector spinae group. In the hook-lying position, the psoas muscle tends to be slackened. This causes the abdominals to play a greater role than if the legs were extended at the knee and hip joints. If the psoas major is to be brought into action during trunk flexion while in the hook-lying position, the feet must be held by some object or by another person.

When the pelvic girdle is moved toward the rib cage (posterior pelvic girdle rotation), a reversal of muscle function in regard to lumbar

Figure 6.1. Abdominal musculature.

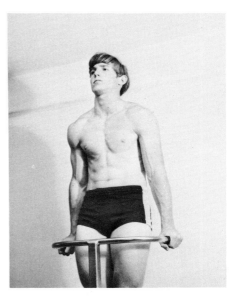

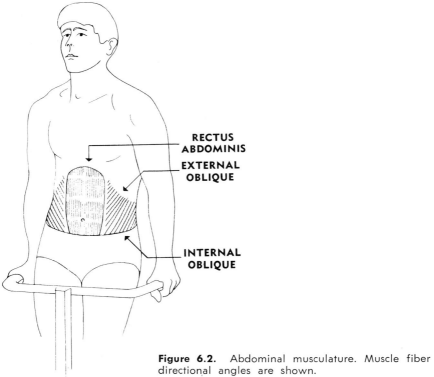

RECTUS
ABDOMINIS

EXTERNAL
OBLIQUE

INTERNAL
OBLIQUE

Figure 6.2. Abdominal musculature. Muscle fiber directional angles are shown.

flexion is seen. As an example, with the performer in a supine position, the legs are moved to a position over the head. The pelvic girdle moves toward the rib cage as lumbar flexion takes place. The moving unit in this example is the pelvic girdle. While doing a hook-lying sit-up, which was described above, the pelvis was relatively fixed. Movement occurred from the proximal to distal attachments of the muscles most involved. In the second example, the rib cage was relatively fixed, and movement was from the distal to the proximal attachment of the muscles most involved. These two examples illustrate the reversal of muscle function.

When analyzing sport activities, the effect of gravity must be considered. Gravitational pull is the major moving force for many motions. For example, trunk flexion from the standing position is performed by the pull of gravity and controlled *eccentrically* by the contracting erector spinae muscle group. The subsequent trunk extension against gravity is performed by the *concentrically* contracting erector spinae muscles. Thus, the abdominal muscle group is not directly involved in trunk flexion performed from the standing position with gravity.

Diagonal flexion can be observed in an athlete who is throwing a ball. Diagonal flexion starts when the overarm throw is initiated. It continues through the full diagonal plane of motion and is completed at the end of the follow-through. Diagonal flexion has occurred within the spinal column, and diagonal adduction has occurred at the glenohumeral joint. Diagonal flexion can occur both right and left. An example of right diagonal flexion was given in the example above. The muscles most involved for right diagonal flexion are the left internal oblique and the right external oblique muscles working together. These muscles in this case, as well as in other examples of sport skills, act as a continuing functional unit. The contralateral muscles for right diagonal flexion are the internal oblique on the right side and the external oblique muscle on the left side. The primary guiding muscles for this action are the erector spinae on the left side and the right side of the rectus abdominis muscle anteriorly. The opposite muscle action would bring about left diagonal flexion.

Right diagonal extension is a movement seen, as an example, when the right-handed quarterback moves his arm, trunk, and pelvis into position preparing to throw. When he does this he places the oblique muscles on stretch just prior to the throw. Right diagonal extension is movement of the right side of the rib cage backward and upward. The muscles most involved for right diagonal extension are the right internal oblique and left external oblique muscles working with the erector spinae muscles contracting concentrically and bilaterally to extend the spine. The contralateral muscles for this movement are the internal oblique muscle on the left and the external oblique muscle on the right. The left half of the rectus abdominis muscle is the main guiding muscle for diagonal extension to the right. Diagonal extension, like diagonal flexion, occurs both right and left. For diagonal extension to the left, the opposite muscles would be involved.

Extension of the lumbar spine against resistance is the direct result of bilateral concentric contraction by the muscles within the erector spinae group (Figures 6.3 and 6.4). In order to have spinal extension

Figure 6.3. Lumbar spine extension.

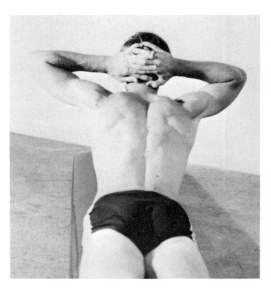

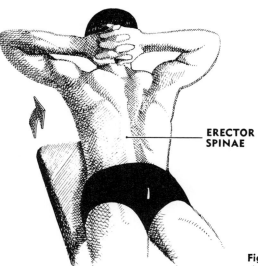

ERECTOR
SPINAE

Figure 6.4 Lumbar spine extension.

through the anteroposterior plane, these muscles must contract equally and bilaterally. The muscles contralateral to lumbar extension are the rectus abdominis, internal oblique, and external oblique muscles. The muscles which serve a guiding function during lumbar extension are the internal and external obliques on the right and left halves of the body. The oblique muscles do this by preventing spinal rotation during concentric contraction of the erector spinae. Extension of the lumbar spine is seen very commonly when there is a jump-ball situation in basketball (Figure 6.5). The extension of the spine follows plantar flexion, knee extension, and hip extension in a sequential fashion.

The muscles most involved in lateral flexion against resistance to the right are the internal and external oblique muscles on the right, right half of the rectus abdominis and the right half of the erector spinae

Figure 6.5. Spinal extension.

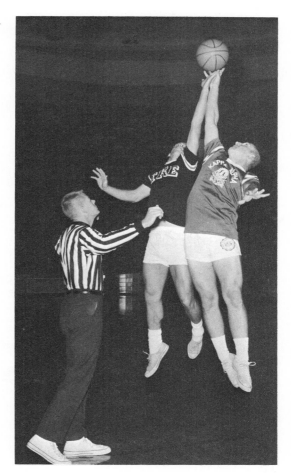

muscles posteriorly (Figures 6.6 and 6.7). These muscles must contract concentrically in order to cause the trunk to move against resistance and gravity to the right. The contralateral muscles for right lateral flexion are the same muscles on the opposite side. The guiding function for right lateral flexion through the lateral plane is provided by the equal balance of force provided by the muscles contracting concentrically anterior and posterior. This balance of force is provided by the muscles most involved for right lateral flexion.

Spinal rotation within the lumbar spine can be best understood by a thorough study of diagonal flexion and diagonal extension. This is

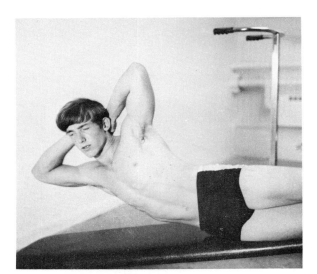

Figure 6.6. Lateral trunk flexion—left.

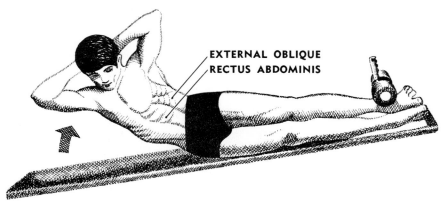

EXTERNAL OBLIQUE
RECTUS ABDOMINIS

Figure 6.7. Lateral trunk flexion—left. (Muscles most involved appear in uppercase letters.)

due to the complexity of superimposing a lateral curve upon an antero-posterior curve, which is seen particularly in the lumbar spinal region. The attention of the physical educator involved in kinesiologic analysis should be centered on the action and interaction between the rib cage and pelvis as functional units instead of being centered on the rotary actions between the vertebrae themselves.

▶ Movements of the Cervical Spine

The vertebrae of the cervical spine are suited to produce a wide range of movement as compared to the larger vertebrae seen in the thoracic and lumbar regions. The movements possible within the cervical spine are flexion, extension, lateral flexion, and rotation. Owing to the relatively small size of the cervical vertebrae, the wide range of motion possible within this area, and the lack of ligamentous support, stability is maintained primarily by the musculature of the neck. Consequently, this region must receive considerable attention when conditioning athletes for contact sports such as soccer and field hockey or an impact sport such as American football.

Flexion of the cervical spine against resistance is performed by both sternocleidomastoid muscles (MMI) contracting concentrically. These two muscles have a spatial relationship anterior to the cervical spine. An example of this type of movement performed by the sternocleido-mastoid is seen when the individual is lying in the supine position and raises the head from the floor. The head moves toward the rib cage through the anteroposterior plane of motion. When the individual is standing and flexes the cervical spine, gravity is a major moving force. The muscles most involved in controlling this action are the erector spinae muscles contracting eccentrically on the posterior aspect of the cervical spine, i. e., the erector spinae are lengthening to allow the head to move forward slowly. The contralateral muscles for cervical flexion against resistance are the erector spinae muscles in the cervical region. The guiding component for cervical flexion is provided by the equal bilateral pull of the contracting sternocleidomastoid muscles. If one sternocleidomastoid muscle were contracting unilaterally, a rotary component would be introduced into the movement.

Extension of the cervical spine against resistance occurs as a result of concentric contraction by the erector spinae muscle group within the cervical region. The spatial relationship of the erector spinae to the cervical vertebrae is posterior. Extension through the anteroposterior range of motion is brought about due to the equal bilateral contraction of the erector spinae muscles on both the right and left halves of the body. The contralateral muscles for cervical extension are the sternocleidomastoid muscles on the anterior aspect of the neck. Guiding action is performed by equal tension within the contracting erector spinae on the right and left halves of the body. If the muscles within the erector spinae group were to contract unilaterally, there would be a rotary action occurring within the cervical spine.

Right and left lateral flexion of the cervical spine occurs through the lateral plane of motion. The muscles most involved in left lateral flexion against resistance are the left sternocleidomastoid and the left muscles within the erector spinae group (Figures 6.8 and 6.9). To move the cervical spine in this direction, these anterior and posterior muscles must contract with equal tension to prevent their rotary functions from occurring. The contralateral muscles for left lateral flexion are the right sternocleidomastoid and the muscles in the right erector spinae group at the cervical level. Here again, guiding function is provided by equal tension within the muscles most involved. Right lateral flexion within the cervical area is a result of contraction by the muscles contralateral to the muscles described for left lateral flexion.

Right cervical rotation is movement of the face toward the right shoulder. The muscles most involved for this action against resistance are the sternocleidomastoid muscle on the left side and the muscles

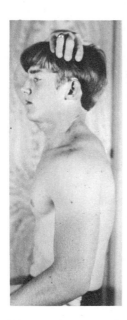

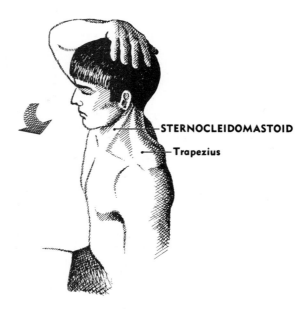

STERNOCLEIDOMASTOID

Trapezius

Figure 6.8. Lateral cervical flexion—left.

Figure 6.9. Lateral cervical flexion—left. (Muscles most involved appear in uppercase letters.)

in the erector spinae group on the right side (Figures 6.10 and 6.11). The contralateral muscles are the right sternocleidomastoid and the muscles within the erector spinae group on the left side in the area of the cervical spine. Again the guiding function is within the muscles most

Figure 6.10. Right cervical rotation.

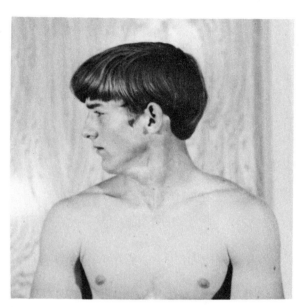

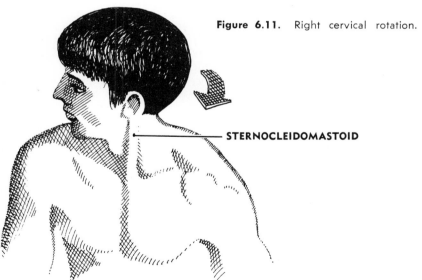

Figure 6.11. Right cervical rotation.

STERNOCLEIDOMASTOID

involved. In this case they eliminate flexion and extension of the cervical spine to bring about the desired rotation. Left rotation of the cervical spine is performed by the muscles contralateral to the muscles described for right cervical spine rotation.

SELECTED REFERENCES

1. BENTELER, A. M. "Change in Tone of the Spinal Muscles in Man." *Sechnor Physiological Journal of the U.S.S.R.* 47:393-98, 1961.
2. COLACHIS, S. C. JR., and OTHERS. "Movement of the Sacroiliac Joint in the Adult Male: Preliminary Report." *Archives of Physical Medicine and Rehabilitation* 44:490-98, September, 1963.
3. DAVIS, P. R. "Posture of the Trunk During the Lifting of Weights." *British Medical Journal* 5114:87-89, 1959.
4. DAVIS, P. R., TROUP, J. D. G., and BURNARD, J. H. "Movements of the Thoracic and Lumbar Spine When Lifting: A Chronocylophotographic Study." *Journal of Anatomy* 99:13-26, January, 1965.
5. DEFIBAUGH, JOSEPH J. "Measurement of Head Motion, Part I: A Review of Methods of Measuring Joint Motion." *Physical Therapy* 44:157-63, March, 1964.
6. ———. "Measurement in Head Motion, Part II: An Experimental Study of Head Motion in Adult Males." *Physical Therapy* 44:163-68, March, 1964.
7. FERLIC, DONALD. "The Range of Motion of the 'Normal' Cervical Spine." *Bulletin of the Johns Hopkins Hospital* 110:59-65, February, 1962.
8. FLINT, M. M. "Effect of Increasing Back and Abdominal Muscle Strength on Low Back Pain," *Research Quarterly* 29:160-71, May, 1958.
9. GOUGH, JOSEPH G., and KOEPKE, GEORGE H. "Electromyographic Determination of Motor Root Levels in Erector Spinae Muscles." *Archives of Physical Medicine and Rehabilitation* 47:9-11, January, 1966.
10. KEAGY, ROBERT D., BRUMLICK, JOEL, and BERGAN, JOHN J. "Direct Electromyography of the Psoas Major Muscle in Man." *Journal of Bone and Joint Surgery* 48-A:1377-82, October, 1966.
11. KOTTKE, FREDERIC J., and MUNDALE, MARTIN O. "Range of Mobility of the Cervical Spine." *Archives of Physical Medicine and Rehabilitation* 40:379-382, September, 1959.
12. LA BAN, MYRON M., and OTHERS. "Electromyographic Study of Function of Iliopsoas Muscle." *Archives of Physical Medicine and Rehabilitation* 46:676-79, October, 1965.
13. MICHELE, ARTHUR A. *Iliopsoas*. Springfield: Charles C Thomas, Publisher, 1962.
14. MORRIS, J. M., BENNER, G., and LUCAS, D. B. "An Electromyographic Study of the Intrinsic Muscles of the Back in Man" *Journal of Anatomy* 96:509-20, October, 1962.
15. NACHEMSON, A. "Electromyographic Studies on the Vertebral Portion of the Psoas Muscle." *Acta Orthopaedica Scandinavica* 37:177-90, Fasc. 2, 1966.
16. PARTRIDGE, MIRIAM J., and WALTERS, C. ETTA. "Participation of the Abdominal Muscles in Various Movements of the Trunk in Man," *Physical Therapy Review* 39:791-800, December, 1959.

17. RAPER, A. JARRELL, and OTHERS. "Scalene and Sternomastoid Muscle Function." *Journal of Applied Physiology* 21:497-502, 1966.
18. SHEFFIELD, F. J. "Electromyographic Study of the Abdominal Muscles in Walking and Other Movements." *American Journal of Physical Medicine* 41:142-147, August, 1962.
19. STEEN, B. "The Function of Certain Neck Muscles in Different Positions of the Head with and without Loading of the Cervical Spine." *Acta Morphologica Neerlando-Scandinavica* VI:301-10, 1966.
20. WALTERS, C. ETTA, and PARTRIDGE, MIRIAM J. "Electromyographic Study of the Differential Action of the Abdominal Muscles During Exercises." *American Journal of Physical Medicine* 36:259-68, October, 1957.

the shoulder girdle
and upper limb

Owing to the lack of bony stability in the shoulder area, the supporting role of the musculature is of paramount concern. Observation in sport of the variety of movements possible within the shoulder area is astonishing. For example, the gymnastics move called the "dislocate," which is performed on the rings, is a remarkable feat substantiating the stability provided by muscles found on the anterior, posterior, medial, and lateral aspects of the shoulder.

The shoulder girdle is composed of the sternoclavicular and acromioclavicular joints, the clavicles, and scapulae. The shoulder girdle is discussed as a separate entity from the shoulder joint. However, the reader must remember that these two areas have a direct, reciprocal relationship to one another, i. e., the movements of the shoulder girdle and shoulder joint cannot be separated when analyzing total shoulder area movements. The separate discussion of the two areas is done herein for the sake of clarity only.

▶ Sternoclavicular Joint

The sternoclavicular joint is one of the most freely movable gliding joints in the body. There is considerable motion allowed because this joint has an interarticular disc. The clavicle moves approximately forty degrees during depression and elevation. It also moves approximately forty degrees anteriorly and posteriorly. From a ligamentous standpoint, the support of the sternoclavicular joint is very strong. There is a fibrocartilage to assist in preventing the upward and medial displacement of the clavicle. This fibrocartilage also absorbs shock received laterally through the acromion process. For example, shock received by a wrestler who is thrown on the "point of his shoulder" is partially absorbed at the sterno-

clavicular joint. The joint receives further support by anterior and posterior sternoclavicular ligments. These ligaments working in conjunction
with the costoclavicular ligament prevent upward and lateral displacement of the clavicle. The interclavicular ligament connects the clavicles.
This ligament prevents the clavicle from being displaced laterally. The
subclavius muscle has a type of "ligamentous function" because it sup-
ports or stabilizes the clavicle. It has an attachment on the first rib and
another attachment on the inferior aspect of the clavicle. Owing to the
relatively small size of the subclavius, it will not be considered as a
muscle most involved for shoulder girdle movements.

▶ Acromioclavicular Joint

The acromioclavicular joint is formed by the articulation between the
clavicle and the scapula. The two sets of scapulae and clavicles form
the shoulder girdle. The acromioclavicular joint is a relatively fixed joint
held together by the superior and inferior acromioclavicular ligaments
as well as the coracoclavicular ligament from below. Due to this ligamentous stability of the bony structures, the movements of the shoulder
girdle are seen functionally within the sternoclavicular joints. There is
very little, if any, muscle support of the acromioclavicular joint because
muscles do not cross it.

▶ Shoulder Girdle Movements

The spatial relationships of the muscles discussed in the shoulder girdle
area are in terms of their positions to the *scapulae* instead of to joints
per se. This approach to spatial relationship differs from other body areas
due to the fact that the scapula is used as a reference point and moving
part instead of a joint.

The muscles most involved in scapular abduction against resistance
are the pectoralis minor and serratus anterior. The contralateral muscles
are the middle fibers of the trapezius and the rhomboid muscles. The
guiding component for scapular abduction is provided by a balance of
forces between the concentrically contracting upper and lower fibers of
the serratus anterior. Complete scapular abduction against resistance is
seen at the highest point in the common push-up. Scapular abduction
against resistance is also observed while doing a bench press. Both
muscles most involved for scapular abduction, the pectoralis minor and
the serratus anterior, have a spatial relationship anterior to the scapula.

The muscles most involved in scapular adduction against resistance
are the middle fibers of the trapezius and the rhomboids. The spatial
relationship of the middle fibers of the trapezius to the scapula tends

to be posterior and medial (Figures 7.1 and 7.2). The spatial relationship of the rhomboids to the scapula is medial, i. e., the rhomboids have attachments on the vertebral border of the scapula and the spinal column. The contralateral muscles for scapular adduction are the pectoralis minor and serratus anterior. The guiding function for this movement is provided

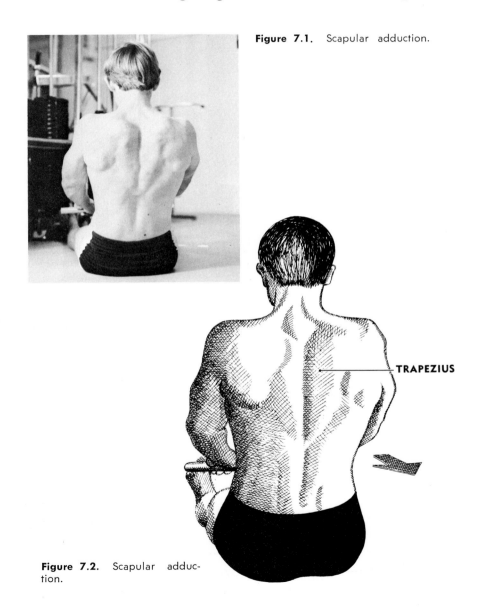

Figure 7.1. Scapular adduction.

TRAPEZIUS

Figure 7.2. Scapular adduction.

by equal tension within the muscles most involved during scapular adduction.

Scapular abduction and adduction can be understood best by study of the relationship between the serratus anterior and rhomboid muscles. These two muscles can be thought of as one myologic unit because they both attach at the vertebral border of the scapulae. When the serratus anterior contracts concentrically against resistance, the rhomboids must contract eccentrically, i. e., they must lengthen while the serratus anterior abducts the scapula. These two muscles maintain a close contact with the rib cage throughout this movement. This action holds the scapulae in a relatively close relationship to the rib cage. Because of the semi-cylindrical shape of the rib cage, it is obvious that the scapulae describes an arc during abduction and adduction. The myologic unit consisting of the serratus anterior and rhomboids also has a relationship with the internal and external oblique muscles. These four muscles are discussed in Chapter 8 in terms of a larger myologic construct known as "the serape effect."

Upward rotation of the scapula involves lateral and upward movement of the inferior angle of the scapula and glenoid fossa. It should be noted that during this movement the anteroposterior axis of the scapula is moving laterally as well as upward during upward rotation. This is due primarily to the fact that motion is allowed within the freely movable sternoclavicular joint. The clavicle actually provides a radius for shoulder girdle movement to occur. It also allows lateral and upward displacement of the scapula.

The position of the upper limbs must be taken under consideration when analyzing or determining the muscles most involved for upward rotation. As pointed out previously, upward rotation of the scapula accompanies any upward, lateral, or diagonal motion of the upper limbs at the glenohumeral joint. The muscles most involved for upward rotation of the scapulae differ in relation to shoulder joint abduction and flexion. This is because of the change in position of the scapula relative to the rib cage when the shoulder joint is abducted or flexed. As can be observed by palpation techniques, the scapulae are in a position closer to the spinal column when the shoulder joint is abducted than when the shoulder joint is flexed. The scapulae are moved away from the vertebral column when the upper limbs are flexed at the shoulder joint. When the upper limbs are flexed at the shoulder joint, the function of the trapezius muscle in upward rotation of the scapula is less because the trapezius is placed in a position of leverage disadvantage for functional concentric contraction and subsequent movement of the scapula into upward rotation.

The muscles most involved in upward rotation of the scapula against resistance while the upper limbs are being abducted are all parts of the trapezius and the lower fibers of the serratus anterior (Figures 7.3 and 7.4). The contralateral muscles for this action are the rhomboids, levator scapulae, and pectoralis minor. The main guiding component comes from

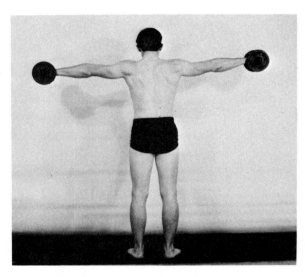

Figure 7.3 Scapular upward rotation concurrent with shoulder joint abduction.

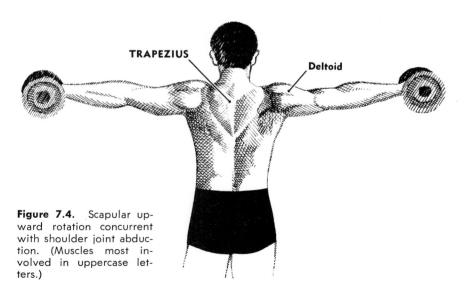

Figure 7.4. Scapular upward rotation concurrent with shoulder joint abduction. (Muscles most involved in uppercase letters.)

the bilateral and equal tension provided by the upper and lower parts of the trapezius. This is primarily due to the fact that the lower fibers of the trapezius exert their force downward on the vertebral base of the scapular spine. Conversely, the upper fibers of the trapezius exert their force upward on the acromion of the spine of the scapulae.

When the upper limbs are flexed at the shoulder joint, the muscle most involved in performing upward rotation of the scapula is the serratus anterior (Figures 7.5 and 7.6). The middle and lower fibers of the trapezius are in a position of disadvantage when flexion occurs at the shoulder joint; however, the upper fibers of the trapezius are involved to a greater extent during upward rotation than the remaining fibers of the trapezius.

Downward rotation of the scapula involves teamwork among muscles located anterior and posterior to the rib cage. The muscles most involved in downward rotation of the scapula against resistance are the rhom-

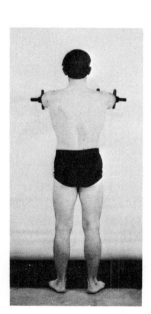

Figure 7.5. Scapular upward rotation concurrent with shoulder joint flexion. Compare the trapezius with Figure 7.3.

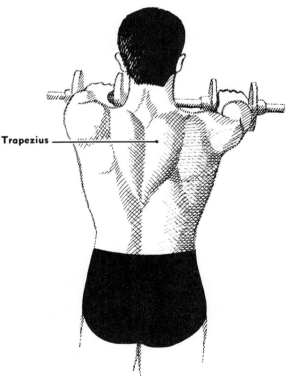

Trapezius

Figure 7.6. Scapular upward rotation concurrent with shoulder joint flexion.

boids, levator scapulae, and pectoralis minor (Figures 7.7 and 7.8). The contralateral muscles for this movement are the trapezius and serratus anterior muscles. The main guiding force in downward rotation of the

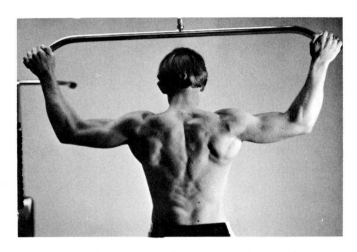

Figure 7.7.   Downward rotation of the scapulae.

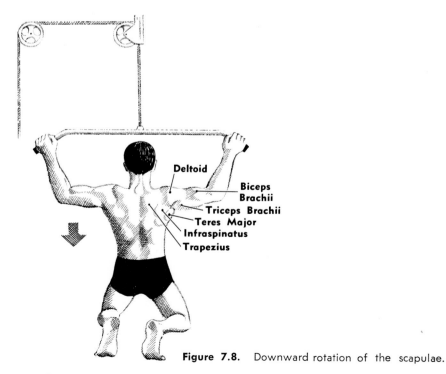

Deltoid

Biceps
Brachii

Triceps Brachii

Teres Major

Infraspinatus

Trapezius

Figure 7.8.   Downward rotation of the scapulae.

scapula is derived from contraction of the lower fibers of the rhomboid major and the levator scapulae.

The muscles most involved in elevation of the scapula against resistance are the levator scapulae, upper trapezius, and rhomboid muscles (Figures 7.9 and 7.10). The contralateral muscles for elevation

Figure 7.9. Elevation.

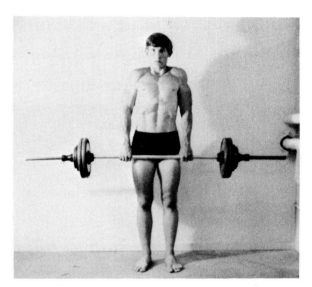

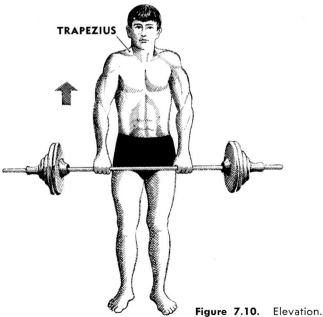

Figure 7.10. Elevation.

of the scapula are the lower trapezius and pectoralis minor. The guiding action for elevation is performed primarily by the levator scapulae and the upper trapezius. These two muscles work together during elevation by counteracting their upward and downward rotary components.

The muscles most involved in depressing the scapula against resistance are the lower trapezius and the pectoralis minor. Here again there is a teamwork function among muscles anterior and posterior to the rib cage. The contralateral muscles for depression of the scapula are the levator scapulae, upper trapezius, and rhomboids. The guiding function is done by equal and bilateral tension within the muscles most involved as they counteract their rotary components.

▶ Shoulder Joint Movements

With the evolution of the human from the quadrupedal to the bipedal stance, a number of changes have taken place within the shoulder joint. When man used the quadrupedal position, the bony structure and alignment of the scapulae and shoulder joint were highly stable to perform the weight-bearing function. However, in the bipedal or non-weight-bearing position, the bony arrangement of the shoulder has changed. The shoulder joint is now free to perform a wide range and variety of motion. The motion demands placed on the muscles surrounding the shoulder joint are largely of a skilled or manipulative nature; consequently, the muscles in the shoulder area tend to be developed below their potential strength in most men and women.

The shoulder joint is classified as an enarthrodial, or ball-and-socket, joint. The term "ball-and-socket" is misleading, especially if the bony structure of the shoulder joint is compared to the hip joint. The bones involved at the shoulder joint are the humerus and scapula. From a bony standpoint, the shoulder joint is not a ball-and-socket type of arrangement because the glenoid fossa does not receive the oval head of the humerus into it. The bony configuration of the glenoid fossa is not deep enough to be considered a natural socket. It becomes a socket by the addition of a ring of fibrocartilage material which, in effect, surrounds the glenoid fossa. This cartilaginous structure is triangular in cross section and is called the glenoid labrum. The glenoid labrum articulates with the head of the humerus. This arrangement of the shoulder joint provides little stability; therefore, the muscle stability at the shoulder joint is more important than in any other major joint of the body.

The articular capsule of the shoulder joint is very loosely oriented. As a result, it adds very little to the overall stability of the joint. Yet it does add to the motility function of the shoulder joint. In the anatomic position, the inferior aspect of the articular capsule actually hangs in folds.

The ligaments in and around the shoulder joint do provide some stability. The major ligamentous support is derived from the coracohumeral ligament. This ligament supplies anterior and superior support from the coracoid process to the head of the humerus. The shoulder joint is also supported ligamentously on its anterior aspect by the transverse ligament.

The integrity of the shoulder joint is maintained primarily by the subscapularis, supraspinatus, infraspinatus, and teres minor muscles. These are called the *rotary cuff muscles,* and they attach to the head of the humerus via their distal attachments. Proximally, the rotary cuff muscles arise from the vertebral border of the scapula. The rotary cuff consists of the four tendons of these muscles as they surround and attach to the tubercles of the humerus. The subscapularis attaches to the lesser tubercle anteriorly; the supraspinatus attaches to the greater tubercle from above, and the infraspinatus and teres minor muscles attach to the greater tubercle posteriorly. Thus, when all four muscles pull together they maintain the head of the humerus within the glenoid labrum. The anterior muscle provides a medial rotation function. The superior muscle works to abduct the arm, and the two posterior muscles serve the function of lateral rotation.

Additional muscle support is provided by the remaining muscles which cross the shoulder joint. The tendon of the long head of the biceps brachii is of particular importance for anterior stability. In fact, anterior stability of the shoulder joint is probably its most important function.

As stated previously, movements at the shoulder joint are accompanied by movements of the shoulder girdle. The shoulder girdle must be stabilized in order for the shoulder joint to move. This is a form of *dynamic stabilization,* i. e., the fixing or stabilizing action of the scapula is continuous throughout the movement involved at the shoulder joint. The scapulae are relatively fixed during the first thirty degrees of shoulder abduction and during the first sixty degrees of shoulder flexion. Beyond that point within these ranges of motion, movement occurs between the shoulder joint and the scapula at a ratio of two degrees to one degree. For example, in arm abduction from thirty degrees to sixty degrees the humerus is moved thirty degrees, and the scapula is moved fifteen degrees. During the fifteen degrees of movement, the muscles moving the scapula continue to perform a dynamic stabilization function for shoulder joint movement.

Further complexity of shoulder joint motions is due to the relationship of the humeral head to the inferior aspect of the acromion process. Several mechanical processes must take place to allow the humeral head to move freely without jamming it into the inferior aspect of the acromion process. For example, when there is concentric contraction taking place within the middle fibers of the deltoid and supraspinatus muscles, force is exerted upon the humerus which has a tendency to lift it vertically. If this force were not counteracted, it would jam the humeral head into the subacromial bursa lying immediately beneath the acromion process. Also, this initial force would greatly delimit the range of motion for arm abduction. In order to prevent the jamming of the head of the humerus against the inferior aspect of the acromion process, the humeral head must be depressed immediately prior to arm abduction or arm flexion. This is performed by the subscapularis, infraspinatus, and teres minor muscles. These muscles working together pull down on the humerus to counteract the force initially established by the deltoid and supraspinatus muscles. By doing this, the depressors of the humeral head provide a counterleverage on the humerus. This allows arm abduction to occur unobstructed. This action of two forces pulling in opposite directions—the supraspinatus and deltoid pulling in one direction against the subscapularis, infraspinatus, and teres minor pulling in another direction—to perform one function is called *force couple action.* (Inman, Saunders, and Abbott, 1944)

There is another movement peculiarity within the shoulder joint which must be given attention. The arm cannot be abducted unless it is laterally rotated. In other words, with the arm held in medial rotation it cannot be abducted throughout 180 degrees of motion. The reason for this phenomenon lies in the fact that lateral rotation is necessary to allow the humeral head to clear the acromion process during abduction of the arm.

The muscles most involved in shoulder flexion against resistance are the muscles found on the anterior aspect of the shoulder joint. These are the anterior deltoid, the upper portion of the pectoralis major, coracobrachialis, and short head of the biceps brachii muscle (Figures 7.11 and 7.12). The contralateral muscles for shoulder joint flexion are the lower fibers of the pectoralis major, latissimus dorsi, teres major, posterior fibers of the deltoid, and long head of the triceps brachii. The guiding action for shoulder flexion against resistance is provided by the medial and lateral rotators of the humerus.

The muscles most involved in shoulder extension against resistance are the lower fibers of the pectoralis major, latissimus dorsi, teres major, posterior fibers of the deltoid, and long head of the triceps brachii. The spatial relationship of these muscles to the shoulder joint is posterior (Figures 7.13 and 7.14). The contralateral muscles for shoulder extension are the anterior deltoid, upper portion of the pectoralis major, coracobrachialis, and short head of the biceps brachii. The guiding muscles for extension at the shoulder joint are the medial and lateral rotators of the humerus.

Figure 7.11. Shoulder joint flexion.

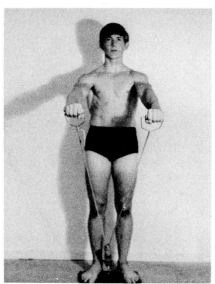

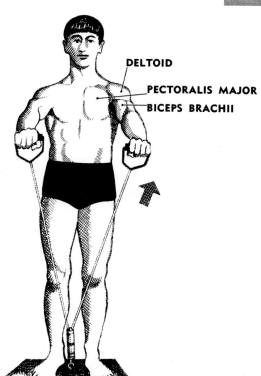

DELTOID

PECTORALIS MAJOR

BICEPS BRACHII

Figure 7.12. Shoulder joint flexion.

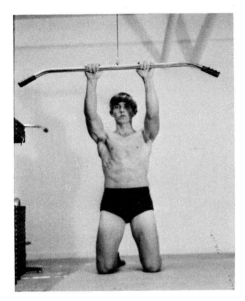

Figure 7.13. Shoulder joint extension.

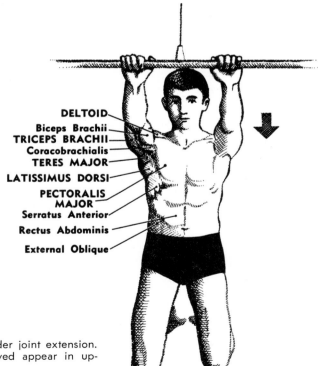

DELTOID
Biceps Brachii
TRICEPS BRACHII
Coracobrachialis
TERES MAJOR
LATISSIMUS DORSI
PECTORALIS
MAJOR
Serratus Anterior
Rectus Abdominis

External Oblique

Figure 7.14. Shoulder joint extension.
(Muscles most involved appear in uppercase letters.)

The deltoid and supraspinatus are the muscles most involved in shoulder joint abduction against resistance (Figures 7.15 and 7.16). The upper fibers of the pectoralis major are also involved in shoulder joint abduction when the arm is raised above the horizontal level. These muscles have a lateral spatial relationship to the shoulder joint. In terms of a mechanical advantage for shoulder joint abduction against resistance, the middle fibers of the deltoid are in the best position to exert force. The contralateral muscles for shoulder joint abduction are the latissimus dorsi, teres major, lower fibers of the pectoralis major, and the long head of the triceps brachii. The guiding action for shoulder joint abduction is provided by the anterior and posterior fibers of the deltoid during shoulder joint abduction.

The latissimus dorsi, teres major, lower fibers of the pectoralis major, and long head of the triceps brachii are the muscles most involved for shoulder joint adduction against resistance. These muscles have a medial

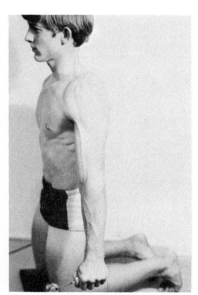

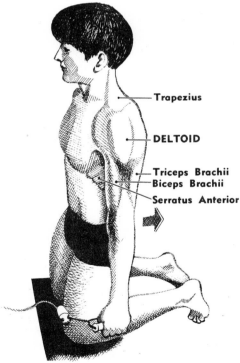

Figure 7.15. Shoulder joint abduction.

Figure 7.16. Shoulder joint abduction. (Muscles most involved appear in uppercase letters.)

spatial relationship to the shoulder joint (Figures 7.17 and 7.18). The contralateral muscles are primarily the deltoid and supraspinatus, although some assistance is provided by the upper fibers of the pectoralis major. The guiding action for shoulder joint adduction is provided by the balance of tension between the long head of the triceps brachii

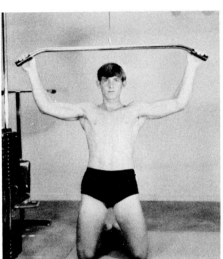

Figure 7.17. Shoulder joint adduction.

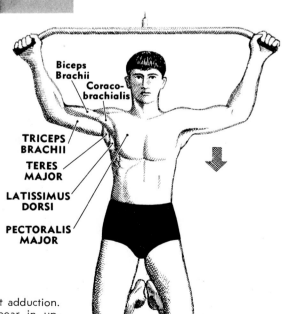

Figure 7.18. Shoulder joint adduction. (Muscles most involved appear in uppercase letters.)

posteriorly and the latissimus dorsi, teres major, and lower fibers of the pectoralis major anteriorly.

The muscles most involved in medial rotation of the humerus against resistance are the teres major, latissimus dorsi, subscapularis, and pectoralis major. The contralateral muscles producing medial rotation are the infraspinatus and teres minor. The guiding component in medial rotation against resistance is supplied by a balance of force between the muscles most involved and the contralateral muscles.

The infraspinatus and teres minor are the muscles most involved in lateral rotation of the humerus against resistance. The contralateral muscles are the teres major, latissmus dorsi, subscapularis, and pectoralis major. The infraspinatus and teres minor have a lateral and posterior spatial relationship to the shoulder joint.

The muscles most involved in horizontal abduction of the shoulder joint against resistance are the middle and posterior fibers of the deltoid, infraspinatus, teres minor, and long head of the triceps brachii muscle (Figures 7.19 and 7.20). The contralateral muscles are the anterior deltoid, pectoralis major, coracobrachialis, and short head of the biceps brachii. The guiding function is performed primarily by the muscles most involved for shoulder joint abduction and adduction.

The muscles most involved in horizontal adduction are the anterior fibers of the deltoid, pectoralis major, coracobrachialis, and short head of the biceps brachii (Figures 7.21 and 7.22). The contralateral muscles are the middle and posterior fibers of the deltoid, infraspinatus, teres minor, and long head of the triceps brachii. The guiding action for horizontal adduction is provided by the abductors and adductors of the shoulder joint.

The muscles most involved in high diagonal abduction are the posterior deltoid, infraspinatus, teres minor, and long head of the triceps brachii. The contralateral muscles are the anterior deltoid, lower fibers of the pectoralis major, coracobrachialis, and short head of the biceps brachii. The guiding action for high diagonal abduction is supplied by the abductors and adductors of the shoulder joint. Lateral rotation of the humerus must accompany high diagonal abduction. Owing to the necessity of this rotary component as a part of high diagonal abduction, the infraspinatus and teres minor muscles play an important role in the overall movement.

The muscles most involved in high diagonal adduction of the shoulder joint are the anterior fibers of the deltoid, lower and middle fibers of the pectoralis major, coracobrachialis, and short head of the biceps brachii (Figures 7.23 and 7.24). The contralateral muscles for this movement are the posterior deltoid, infraspinatus, teres minor, and long head of the triceps brachii. The guiding action is provided by the medial and lateral rotators of the humerus. High diagonal adduction at the shoulder

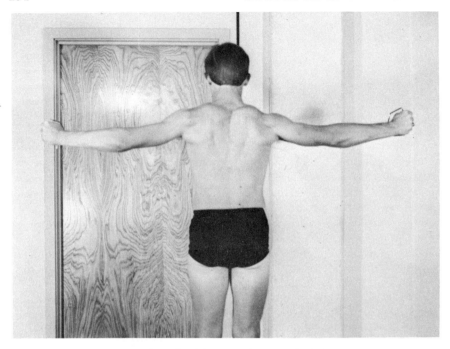

Figure 7.19. Shoulder joint horizontal abduction.

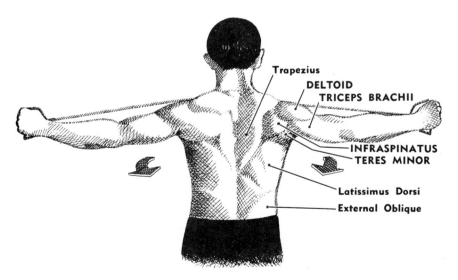

Figure 7.20. Shoulder joint horizontal abduction. (Muscles most involved appear in uppercase letters.)

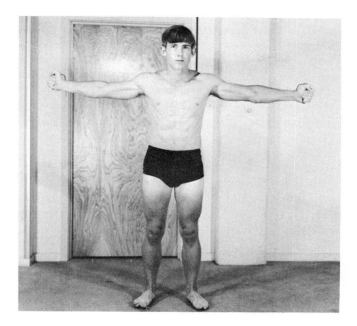

Figure 7.21. Shoulder joint horizontal adduction.

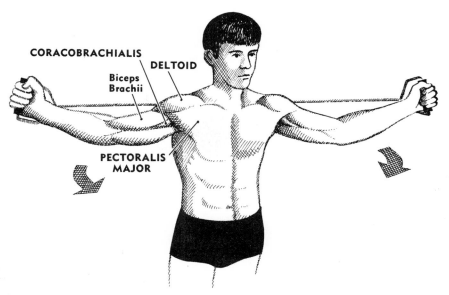

Figure 7.22. Shoulder joint horizontal adduction. (Muscles most involved appear in uppercase letters.)

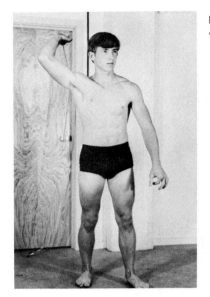

Figure 7.23. High shoulder joint diagonal adduction.

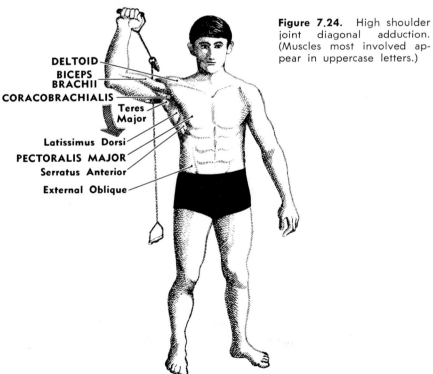

Figure 7.24. High shoulder joint diagonal adduction. (Muscles most involved appear in uppercase letters.)

DELTOID
BICEPS BRACHII
CORACOBRACHIALIS
Teres Major
Latissimus Dorsi
PECTORALIS MAJOR
Serratus Anterior
External Oblique

joint, as commonly seen in ballistic action of the upper limbs during sport performances, is usually accompanied by medial rotation of the humerus. Medial rotation during high diagonal adduction involves the teres major, latissimus dorsi, and subscapularis muscles. These muscles provide an additive factor to the summation of internal forces sequentially transferred to the elbow and wrist joints and to the object to be thrown.

The muscles most involved in low diagonal abduction of the shoulder joint against resistance are the posterior fibers of the deltoid, infraspinatus, teres minor, and long head of the triceps brachii. The contralateral muscles for low diagonal abduction are the anterior fibers of the deltoid, upper fibers of the pectoralis major, coracobrachialis, and short head of the biceps brachii. Guiding low diagonal abduction are the abductors and adductors of the shoulder joint. The movement of low diagonal abduction is commonly seen when the right-handed baseball hitter swings at a pitch low and away from him. The left upper limb of the right-handed hitter is diagonally abducted through the low diagonal plane of motion at the shoulder joint.

The muscles most involved in low diagonal adduction against resistance at the shoulder joint are the anterior fibers of the deltoid, upper fibers of the pectoralis major, coracobrachialis, and short head of the biceps brachii. The contralateral muscles for low diagonal adduction are the posterior fibers of the deltoid, infraspinatus, teres minor, and long head of the triceps brachii. The guiding function is provided by the abductors and adductors of the shoulder joint. Low diagonal adduction at the shoulder joint is seen during the final phase of the discus throw.

▶ Elbow Joint Movements

The elbow articulation is composed of three bones: the humerus, ulna, and radius. On the medial aspect, the humerus articulates with the ulna, and on the lateral side the humerus articulates with the radius. The bony articulation between the humerus and ulna tends to be stable. On the other hand, the articulation between the humerus and the radius lacks bony stability. The hinge arrangement of the elbow joint occurs at the articulation between the humerus and ulna. This deep articulation provides considerable bony stability. It also is a limiting factor as far as motion is concerned because it only allows flexion and extension to occur within the elbow joint.

The ligamentous support of the elbow joint is provided by three ligaments. The lateral support is provided by the radial collateral ligament. Medial support is by the ulnar collateral ligament. The annular ligament maintains the position of the radius at its proximal head.

Hyperextension of the elbow is prevented in the normal upper limb primarily by the proximal end of the ulna contacting the olecranon fossa on the distal aspect of the humerus. Flexion, on the other hand, is limited by the size of the muscle mass on the anterior aspect of the proximal portion of the upper limb.

The elbow is well supplied with muscle to add stability to the joint. Anterior stability is provided by the biceps brachii, brachialis, and brachioradialis muscles. The major posterior stability is from the triceps brachii muscle. This muscular support is further enhanced by the proximal attachments of muscles on the medial and lateral epicondyles of the humerus. The muscles arising from the medial epicondyle are the flexor carpi radialis, palmaris longus, flexor carpi ulnaris, pronator teres, and flexor digitorum superficialis. The lateral stability is provided by the extensor carpi radialis longus, extensor carpi radialis brevis, extensor carpi ulnaris, humeral head of the supinator, extensor digitorum, and extensor digiti minimi. With the exception of the pronator teres and

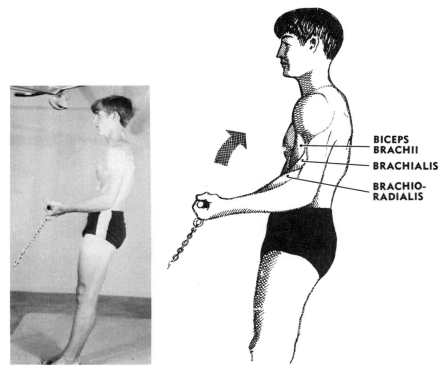

BICEPS
BRACHII

BRACHIALIS

BRACHIO-
RADIALIS

Figure 7.25. Elbow flexion.

Figure 7.26. Elbow flexion. (Muscles most involved appear in uppercase letters.)

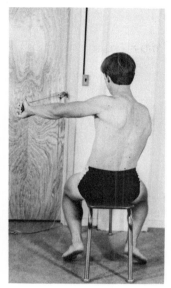

Figure 7.27. Elbow extension.

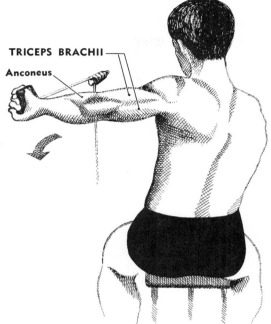

Figure 7.28. Elbow extension. (Muscles most
involved appear in uppercase letters.)

supinator muscles, these multiarticular muscles also act at the wrist and
within the hand.

The muscles most involved in elbow flexion against resistance are
the biceps brachii, brachialis, and brachioradialis (Figures 7.25 and 7.26).
The contralateral muscle is the triceps brachii. No guiding muscles are
needed for elbow flexion owing to the uniaxial structure of the elbow
joint.

The triceps brachii is the muscle most involved in elbow extension
against resistance (Figures 7.27 and 7.28). The contralateral muscles
are the biceps brachii, brachialis, and brachioradialis. Because of the
bony configuration of the elbow joint, a guiding function is not required
for elbow extension.

▶ Radio-Ulnar Joint Movements

There are two bony articulations within the radio-ulnar joint *per se.*
These are described as the articulations between the radius and ulna

proximally and distally. The radius and ulna articulate with each other proximally when the head of the radius contacts the radial notch of the ulna. Distally, the head of the ulna articulates with the ulnar notch of the radius. This is an unstable bony arrangement. Between these two proximal and distal articulations, the two bones do not come into direct contact with each other. Their relative relationship is maintained by means of an interosseous membrane. This interosseous membrane lies between the ulna and radius attaching these two bones together throughout their total length.

Ligamentous support of the radio-ulnar joints is provided by the annular ligament. The interosseous membrane also provides some support of the joint medially. There are anterior and posterior ligaments distally, which are called the volar radio-ulnar ligament and dorsal radioulnar ligament respectively. The ligamentous support within these joints must be relatively free to allow the bones to articulate with each other throughout the movements of pronation and supination.

The muscles most involved in pronation against resistance are the pronator teres and pronator quadratus. These muscles have an anterior spatial relationship to the radio-ulnar joints (Figures 7.29 and 7.30). The pronator teres is located proximally, and the pronator quadratus is located distally on the forearm. The contralateral muscles for pronation are the biceps brachii and supinator.

The muscles most involved in supination against resistance are the biceps brachii and supinator. The line of pull of the supinator is from the lateral aspect of the humerus around to the posterior portion of the radius. The line of pull of the biceps brachii for supination is posterior to anterior, since its distal attachment is on the radial tuberosity. The tendon of the biceps brachii wraps around the head of the radius during pronation; consequently, when the biceps brachii contracts concentrically to perform supination against resistance, the tendon of the biceps brachii literally "unwinds" and rotates the radius laterally around its longitudinal axis. The contralateral muscles for supination are the pronator teres and pronator quadratus.

After the initiation of elbow flexion against resistance, the brachioradialis must be considered as a muscle most involved for both pronation and supination. From either the position of supination or pronation, the brachioradialis will tend to pronate or supinate the radio-ulnar joint to the mid-position when the elbow is flexed. Consequently, during kinesiologic analysis when the elbow is flexed, the brachioradialis must be considered as one of the muscles most involved for pronation or supination if these movements occur. The mid-position referred to above is halfway between pronation and supination.

Figure 7.29. Pronation.

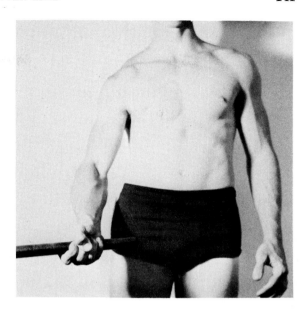

Figure 7.30. Pronation. (Muscles most involved appear in uppercase letters.)

BRACHIORADIALIS——

PRONATOR TERES——

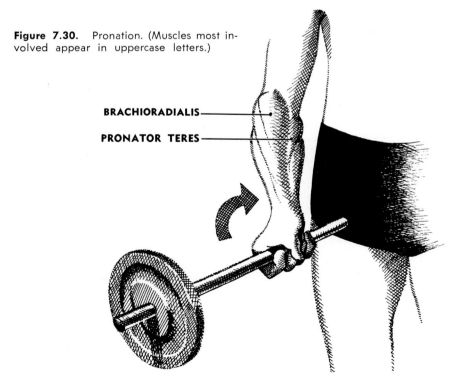

Due to the limited number of movements possible within the radio-ulnar joint, guiding force is not required for pronation or supination. This same mechanism was observed in the elbow joint.

▶ The Wrist Joint Movements

The wrist joint consists of the articulations between the distal end of the radius, navicular, lunate, and triangular carpal bones. From a bony standpoint, the wrist is a stable structure. The three carpal bones are received into the radius in a deep ovoid structure. This articulation allows flexion, extension, radial flexion, and ulnar flexion. The latter two movements can be considered as abduction and adduction movements; consequently, circumduction is also possible at the wrist joint.

The wrist is stable due to the arrangement of the ligaments surrounding the joint. There is anterior, posterior, lateral, and medial ligamentous support. Anterior ligamentous support is maintained by the volar radiocarpal ligament. Posterior support is offered by the dorsal radiocarpal ligament. The ulnar collateral ligament provides support medially, and the radiocarpal ligament maintains support laterally.

The wrist joint is amply provided with muscular support. There are fifteen extrinsic muscles of the hand located on the anterior, posterior, medial, and lateral aspects of the wrist joint. All of these muscles provide muscular stability. The discussion below is delimited to include the extrinsic muscles of the hand. The muscles located entirely within the hand, the intrinsic muscles, are not included within this text.

The muscles most involved in wrist flexion are the flexor carpi radialis, flexor carpi ulnaris, palmaris longus, flexor digitorum superficialis, flexor digitorum profundus, and flexor pollicis longus. All of these muscles have an anterior spatial relationship to the wrist joint. The contralateral muscles for wrist flexion are the muscles located on the posterior aspect of the wrist. These contralateral muscles are the extensor carpi radialis longus, extensor carpi radialis brevis, extensor carpi ulnaris, extensor digitorum, extensor indicis, extensor digiti minimi, extensor pollicis longus, and extensor pollicis brevis. The guiding action is provided by the radial and ulnar flexors of the wrist.

The muscles most involved in wrist extension are the extensor carpi radialis longus, extensor carpi radialis brevis, extensor carpi ulnaris, extensor digitorum, extensor indicis, extensor digiti minimi, extensor pollicis longus, and extensor pollicis brevis. These muscles all have a posterior spatial relationship to the wrist joint. The contralateral muscles for wrist extension are the flexor carpi radialis, flexor carpi ulnaris, palmaris longus, flexor digitorum superficialis, flexor digitorum profundus, and flexor pollicis longus. The guiding force for wrist extension is supplied by the radial and ulnar flexors of the wrist.

The muscles most involved in radial flexion are the flexor carpi radialis, extensor carpi radialis longus, extensor carpi radialis brevis, extensor pollicis brevis, and abductor pollicis longus. These muscles have a lateral spatial relationship to the wrist joint (Figures 7.31 and 7.32).

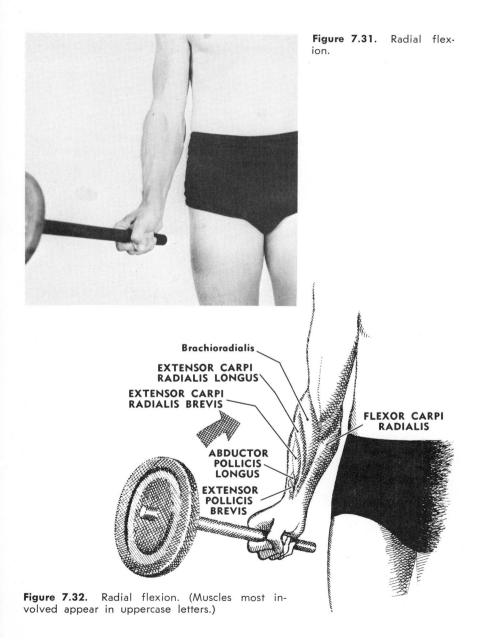

Figure 7.31. Radial flexion.

Brachioradialis

EXTENSOR CARPI RADIALIS LONGUS

EXTENSOR CARPI RADIALIS BREVIS

FLEXOR CARPI RADIALIS

ABDUCTOR POLLICIS LONGUS

EXTENSOR POLLICIS BREVIS

Figure 7.32. Radial flexion. (Muscles most involved appear in uppercase letters.)

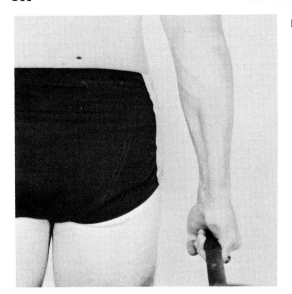

Figure 7.33. Ulnar flexion.

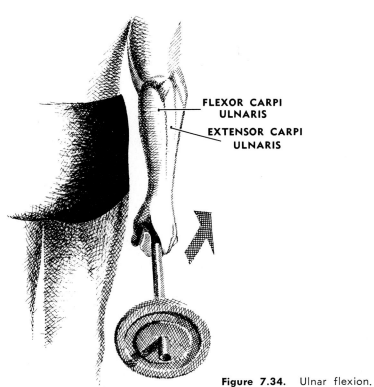

FLEXOR CARPI
ULNARIS

EXTENSOR CARPI
ULNARIS

Figure 7.34. Ulnar flexion.

The contralateral muscles for radial flexion are the flexor carpi ulnaris and extensor carpi ulnaris. The guiding function for radial flexion is provided by the flexor carpi radialis on the anterior aspect of the wrist and by the extensor carpi radialis longus, extensor carpi radialis brevis, extensor pollicis brevis, and abductor pollicis longus on the posterior side.

The muscles most involved in ulnar flexion against resistance are the flexor carpi ulnaris and extensor carpi ulnaris (Figures 7.33 and 7.34). The contralateral muscles for ulnar flexion are the flexor carpi radialis, extensor carpi radialis longus, extensor carpi radialis brevis, extensor pollicis brevis, and abductor pollicis longus. Guiding forces for ulnar flexion are provided by the two muscles most involved. The flexor carpi ulnaris provides a guiding function anteriorly, and the extensor carpi ulnaris offers a guiding function posteriorly.

▶ Metacarpophalangeal and Interphalangeal Joint Movements

The discussion of the extrinsic muscles of the hand is limited to flexion and extension at the metacarpophalangeal and interphalangeal joints. It is recognized, of course, that some of these extrinsic muscles are also involved with the intrinsic muscles of the hand to perform abduction and adduction of the digits as well as extension of the interphalangeal joints.

The muscles most involved in metacarpophalangeal and interphalangeal flexion against resistance are the flexor digitorum profundus, flexor digitorum superficialis, and flexor pollicis longus. These muscles have a spatial relationship anterior to the joint, i. e., they are located on the volar surface of the hand. The contralateral muscles for metacarpophalangeal and interphalangel flexion are the extensor digitorum, extensor indicis, extensor digiti minimi, extensor pollicis longus, and extensor pollicis brevis. Guiding action within this area must be considered in terms of the metacarpophalangeal joints only. The guiding force for flexion at the metacarpophalangeal joints of the fingers is provided by the abductors and adductors of the metacarpophalangeal joints. The metacarpophalangeal joint of the thumb does not require guiding action because it only allows flexion and extension.

The muscles most involved in metacarpophalangeal and interphalangeal joint extension are the extensor digitorum, extensor indicis, extensor digiti minimi, extensor pollicis longus, and extensor pollicis brevis. It is essential for extension within the interphalangeal joints that these extrinsic muscles work with the intrinsic muscles of the hand. The extrinsic muscles have a posterior spatial relationship to the wrist joint and to the metacarpophalangeal and interphalangeal joints. The contralateral muscles for metacarpophalangeal and interphalangeal joint extension are the flexor digitorum profundus, flexor digitorum superficialis, and the flexor pollicis longus. Guiding action is performed by the abductors and adductors of the metacarpophalangeal joints of the four fingers as described above.

SELECTED REFERENCES

1. BASMAJIAN, JOHN V., and TRAVILL, ANTHONY. "Electromyography of the Pronator Muscles in the Forearm." *Anatomical Record* 139: 45-49, 1961.
2. BEARN, J. G. "An Electromyographic Study of the Trapezius, Deltoid, Pectoralis Major, Biceps and Triceps Muscles During Static Loading of the Upper Limb." *Anatomical Record* 140:103-107, June, 1961.
3. ———. "Function of Certain Shoulder Muscles in Posture and in Holding Weights." *Annals of Physical Medicine* 6:100-104, August, 1961.
4. CLARKE, H. HARRISON, and OTHERS. "Conditions for Optimum Work Output in Elbow Flexion, Shoulder Flexion and Grip Ergography." *Archives of Physical Medicine and Rehabilitation* 39:475-81, August, 1958.
5. COPPOCK, D. E. "Relationship of Tightness of Pectoral Muscles to Round Shoulders in College Women." *Research Quarterly* 29:139-45, May, 1958.
6. DEMPSTER, WILFRID T. "Mechanisms of Shoulder Movement." *Archives of Physical Medicine and Rehabilitation* 46:49-70, January, 1965.
7. DeSOUSA, O. MACHADO, and OTHERS. "Electromyographic Study of the Brachioradialis Muscle." *Anatomical Record* 139:125-131, 1961.
8. DIVILEY, REX L., and MEYER, PAUL W. "Baseball Shoulder." *The Journal of the American Medical Association* 171:12:1959-61, November 21, 1959.
9. DUVALL, E. N. "Critical Analysis of Divergent Views of Movement at the Shoulder Joint." *Archives of Physical Medicine* 36:149-154, 1955.
10. INMAN, VERNE T., SAUNDERS, J. B. DeC.M., and ABBOTT, LEROY C. "Observations on the Function of the Shoulder Joint." *Journal of Bone and Joint Surgery* 26:1-30, 1944.
11. LITTLE, ANN D., and LEHMKUHL, DON. "Elbow Extension Force." *Physical Therapy* 46:7-17, January, 1966.
12. LONG, CHARLES, and BROWN, MARY ELEANOR. "Electromyographic Kinesiology of the Hand: Muscles Moving the Long Finger." *Journal of Bone and Joint Surgery* 46A:1683-1705, December, 1964.
13. MARMOR, L., and OTHERS. "Pectoralis Major Muscle." *Journal of Bone and Joint Surgery* 43A:81-87, 1961.
14. McCLOY, C. H. "The Apparent Importance of Arm Strength in Athletics." *Research Quarterly* 5:3, March, 1934.
15. McCRAW, LYNN W. "Effects of Variations of Forearm Positions in Elbow Flexion." *Research Quarterly* 35:504-510, December, 1964.
16. McFARLAND, G. B., KRUSEN, U. L., and WEATHERBY, H. T. "Kinesiology of Selected Muscles Acting on the Wrist: Electromyographic Study." *Archives of Physical Medicine and Rehabilitation* 43:165-171, April, 1962.
17. NELSON, RICHARD C., and FAHRNEY, RICHARD A. "Relationship Between Strength and Speed of Elbow Flexion." *Research Quarterly* 36:455-463, December, 1965.
18. PROVINS, K. A., and SALTER, N. "Maximum Torque Exerted About the Elbow Joint." *Journal of Applied Physiology* 7:393-398, 1955.

19. RAMSEY, ROBERT W., and OTHERS. "An Analysis of Alternating Movements of the Human Arm." *Federation Proceedings* 19:254, March, 1960.
20. RASCH, PHILIP J. "Effect of the Position of Forearm on Strength of Elbow Flexion." *Research Quarterly* 27:333-337, 1956.
21. RAY, ROBERT D., JOHNSON, ROBERT J., and JAMESON, ROBERT M. "Rotation of the Forearm." *Journal of Bone and Joint Surgery* 33-A:993-996, 1951.
22. REEDER, THELMA. "Electromyographic Study of the Latissimus Dorsi Muscle." *Journal of the American Physical Therapy Association* 43:165-172, March, 1963.
23. SCHENKER, A. W. "Finger Joint Motion: A New, Rapid, Accurate Method of Measurement." *Military Medicine* 131:22-29, January, 1966.
24. SIGERSETH, P. O., and McCLOY, C. H. "Electromyographic Study of Selected Muscles Involved in Movements of Upper Arm at the Scapulohumeral Joint." *Research Quarterly* 27:409, December, 1956.
25. SILLS, FRANK D., and OLSON, A. L. "Action Potentials in the Unexercised Arm When Opposite Arm Is Exercised." *Research Quarterly* 29:213-221, May, 1958.
26. SLAUGHTER, DUANE R. "Electromyographic Studies of Arm Movements." *Research Quarterly* 30:326-337, October, 1959.
27. SULLIVAN, W. E., and OTHERS. "Electromyographic Studies of M. Biceps Brachii During Normal Voluntary Movement at the Elbow." *Anatomical Record* 107:243-251, 1950.
28. TAYLOR, CRAIG L., and SCHWARTZ, ROBERT J. "The Anatomy and Mechanics of the Human Hand." *Artificial Limbs* 2:22-35, 1955.
29. TRAVILL, A. A. "Study of the Extensor Apparatus of the Forearm." *Anatomical Review* 144:373-376, 1962.
30. TRAVILL, ANTHONY, and BASMAJIAN, JOHN V. "Electromyography of the Supinators of the Forearm." *Anatomical Record* 139:557-560, 1960.
31. VAN LINGE, B., and MULDER, J. O. "Function of the Supraspinatus Muscle and Its Relation to the Supraspinatus Syndrome." *Journal of Bone and Joint Surgery* 45B:750-754, 1963.
32. WEATHERSBY, HAL T., and OTHERS. "The Kinesiology of Muscles of the Thumb: An Electromyographic Study." *Archives of Physical Medicine and Rehabilitation* 44:321-326, June, 1963.
33. WHITLEY, JIM D., and SMITH, LEON E. "Measurement of Strength of Adduction of the Arm in Various Positions." *Archives of Physical Medicine and Rehabilitation* 45:326-328, July, 1964.
34. WIEDENBAUER, M. M., and MORTENSEN, O. A. "An Electromyographic Study of the Trapezius Muscle." *American Journal of Physical Medicine* 31:363-373, 1952.
35. YAMSHON, L. J., and BIERMAN, W. "Kinesiologic Electromyography, I. The Trapezius." *Archives of Physical Medicine* 24:647-651, 1948.
36. ———. "Kinesiologic Electromyography, III. The Deltoid." *Archives of Physical Medicine* 30:286-289, 1949.

antigravity musculature

Aggregate muscle action refers to the general concept that muscles work in groups rather than working independently to achieve a given joint action. Muscles have two major functions: (1) to pull on the bony levers to cause motion at articulations and (2) to maintain the body in a variety of positions both moving and relatively stationary against the pull of gravity. The first function of muscles was discussed in Chapters 4 through 7. The second function is discussed in this chapter.

The term "aggregate muscle action" is used to imply the muscular teamwork which is necessary at joints in order to perform a specific movement. There is also seen within the human organism another type of teamwork between or among muscles within muscle groups. One of these functions involves the maintenance of the upright, or bipedal, position. This requires a considerable amount of integrated activity among several large and important muscle groups of the body. These muscle groups are primarily the extensors of the major joints of the body. The individual in a normal upright stance will exhibit a very slight amount of flexion at the ankle, knee, and hip joints. Furthermore, there is also a slight forward lean of the trunk in the normal upright stance. There are at least two major reasons for these tendencies toward flexion. Flexion occurs due to the (1) anatomic or bony structure of the joints at the ankle, knee, hip, and spinal column and (2) effect of the downward pull of gravity on these joints. Furthermore, the slight amount of flexion observed is necessary for subsequent movements on the part of the individual—this is sometimes called the "position of readiness." What appears to be static stabilization occurring at the major joints of the body is in reality dynamic stabilization because the body is in constant motion as it reacts to the force of gravity.

It is believed by some physical educators that there is a standard by which posture can be measured for all individuals. This so-called standard is based largely upon aesthetics. Historically, it can be traced to studies done in Germany during the nineteenth century by Braune and Fischer. Braune and Fischer calculated the center of gravity of the total body and its limbs by making calculations on two frozen, dissected cadavers. They compared their findings with a photograph of a living soldier, and they observed that there was considerable similarity between their cadaver findings and the posture of the soldier. Consequently, they stated that the original position of their cadavers could be considered normal. Unfortunately, some physical educators erroneously interpreted the findings of Braune and Fischer to mean that all people considered to be normal from a postural standpoint should conform to the "Braune and Fischer Measurements." Thus, the measurements of Braune and Fischer have become "posture standards" in some physical education programs. (Rasch and Burke, 1967)

Metheny's comments exemplify current trends and practices—there should be no rigid posture standards for all people. She emphasized that each person has one body and the individual must make the most of it. Posture is a highly individual matter. (Metheny, 1952)

Although it is obvious that "good posture" is desirable from an aesthetic standpoint, it does not follow that the individual with good posture will be a better athlete because of his posture. The mature athlete tends to have a posture which is related to his particular sport if he has trained for years to become expert at his specific position or event. The reason for this phenomenon is the fact that the body tends to adjust or adapt to the various stresses or demands imposed upon it as a result of prolonged muscular activity. Wallis and Logan have called this the *SAID Principle*: SAID is an acronym for Specific Adaptations to Imposed Demands. (Wallis and Logan, 1964) The large variety of postures observed among athletes is due to their specific bodily adaptations to imposed demands which result in changes in strength, local muscular endurance, cardiovascular endurance, flexibility, and skill requirements of their various individual sport positions or events. These "postural deviations" from so-called ideal posture standards seen in the athlete as a result of adaptations to imposed demands are not pathalogic in nature. As a matter of fact, these specific changes at times tend to enhance the skill level of the performer at his position. On the other hand, there are times within the "normal individual" or nonathlete when such deviations may be contraindicated.

The antigravity muscles are the most important muscle groups which make possible the maintenance of body postures in sport, exercise, and dance situations. The antigravity musculature must be considered both from anteroposterior as well as lateral standpoints. Because of the body's tendency toward flexion, as noted above, the anteroposterior antigravity muscles must be considered most important. *Anteroposterior antigravity muscles serve as a form of "foundation" for the superimposition of skilled movements.* Therefore, all of the anteroposterior antigravity muscles must be given prime consideration in conditioning and/or weight-training programs for performers of both sexes.

There are four major groups of muscles which work together to keep the body in the bipedal position against gravity. These are the triceps surae, quadriceps femoris muscle group, the gluteus maximus and erector spinae muscle group (Figure 8.1). The rectus abdominis muscle is also considered to be an antigravity muscle from a reflex standpoint. The triceps surae muscles, the gastrocnemius and soleus, perform an antigravity function at the ankle joint through plantar flexion. However, it must be noted that the soleus provides most force for this because the gastrocnemius has a function at the knee as well as at the ankle. At the knee, the quadriceps femoris muscle group acts as a functional unit to extend the knee against gravity. Within this muscle group, the three vasti muscles are primarily involved in the antigravity function because the rectus femoris is a biarticular muscle acting at the hip as well as the knee. At the hip joint, the antigravity function is performed primarily by the gluteus maximus muscle. Extension of the spine is maintained primarily by the erector spinae group contracting equally and bilaterally. This muscle group is assisted in the antigravity function by the deep posterior spinal muscles.

During the contraction of the erector spinae muscles and the deep posterior spinal group while maintaining the spinal column in the antigravity position, the rectus abdominis contracts reflexly to maintain a relatively constant position between the rib cage and pelvic girdle. Thus, the rectus abdominis also serves an anteroposterior antigravity function.

Playing an important antigravity function, but perhaps less important than anteroposterior antigravity musculature, is the lateral antigravity musculature (Figure 8.2). These antigravity muscles perform their movements at the ankle, hip, lumbar, and cervical spinal areas. Their movements at the ankle are eversion and inversion. The knee, owing to its structure, has lateral stability provided by the anteroposterior musculature. The lateral antigravity muscle groups of the hip are the abductors and adductors. Lateral stability of the lumbar and cervical spine areas is performed by the lateral flexors of the spine. Both the rectus abdominis and the erector spinae serve as lateral flexors of the lumbar spine; consequently, they serve a dual role as lateral and anteroposterior antigravity muscles. The erector spinae, in conjunction with the sternocleidomastoid, serve an antigravity role within the cervical spine.

Figure 8.1. Anteroposterior antigravity musculature.

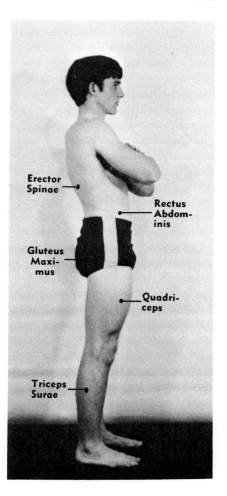

Figure 8.2. Lateral antigravity musculature.

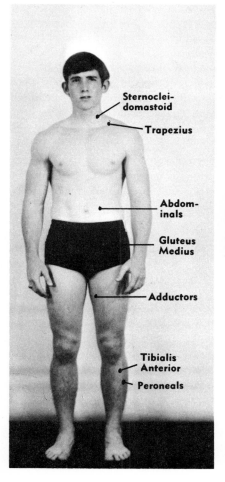

When considering total body movements in relation to the earth, the terms "vertical" and "horizontal" are used because of the downward pull of gravity. Bodily position must be described as being either vertical, horizontal, or in a position between these two extremes in relation to the surface of the earth.

When the body is in a vertical position, the anteroposterior and lateral antigravity groups are working together to maintain the position of extension at the joints involved. In any vertical position relative to the earth's surface, the antigravity musculature is mainly involved to maintain extension within the various joints. During a sport skill or exercise, any movement from the vertical to the horizontal position requires an interaction of the antigravity muscles with other muscle groups to maintain the desired position against the pull of gravity to complete the sport skill or exercise volitionally initiated. An example of this change of position from the vertical to the horizontal is exemplified when the gymnast, working on the parallel bars, moves from a vertical handstand to a full horizontal body lever. It is obvious that during kinesiologic analyses a consideration of gravitational pull must be taken into account when the body is moving through space. Movement problems in outer space are considerably different from movements through space on or near earth. Also, movements within inner space, aquatic movements, are considerably different from movements on land or in outer space. In all three of these situations there is a distinctly different problem as far as gravity is concerned. The physical educator must be primarily concerned about movement on or near the surface of the earth or within water. Some physical educators, such as Dr. Gordon Wells, of North American Space Research, and Dr. William Pierson, at Lockheed, are concerned with movement and exercise problems in outer space. There is no doubt that study of movement in outer space will contribute to man's knowledge of movement on land or in water.

Selected References

1. Agan, T., and others. "A Method of Measuring Postural Attitudes." *Ergonomics* 8:207-222, April, 1965.
2. Basmajian, J. V. "Weight Bearing by Ligaments and Muscles." *Canadian Journal of Surgery* 4:166-170, 1961.
3. ———. "Man's Posture." *Archives of Physical Medicine* 46:26-36, 1965.
4. Fenn, W. O. "Work Against Gravity and Work Due to Velocity Changes in Running." *American Journal of Physiology* 95:433-462, 1930.
5. Flint, M. Marilyn, and Diehl, Bobbie. "Influence of Abdominal Strength, Back Extensor Strength and Trunk Strength Balance Upon Antero-Postero Alignment of Elementary School Girls." *Research Quarterly* 32:490-498, December, 1961.

6. GANSLEN, RICHARD V. "Do Athletes Defy the Law of Gravity?" *Sports College News*, October, 1955.

7. GERSTEN, J. W. "Mechanics of Body Elevation by Gastrocnemius-Soleus Contraction." *American Journal of Physical Medicine* 35:12-16, 1956.

8. GROMBACK, J. V. "The Gravity Factor in World Athletics." *Amateur Athlete* 31:24-25, 1960.

9. HALLEN, L. G., and LINDAHL, O. "The Lateral Stability of the Knee Joint." *Acta Orthopaedica Scandinavica* 36:179-191, 1965.

10. HELLEBRANDT, F. A., and FRANSUN, E. B. "Physiological Study of the Vertical Stance of Man." *Physiological Review* 23:220, 1943.

11. HOUTZ, S. J., LEBOW, M. J., and BEYER, F. R. "Effect of Posture on Strength of the Knee Flexor and Extensor Muscles." *Journal of Applied Physiology* 11:475-480, November, 1957.

12. MARGARIA, R., and CAVAGNA, G. A. "Human Locomotion in Subgravity." *Aerospace Medicine* 35:1140-1146, December, 1964.

13. METHENY, ELEANOR. *Body Dynamics*. New York: McGraw-Hill, Inc., 1952.

14. PORTNOY, H., and MORIN, F. "Electromyographic Study of Postural Muscles in Various Positions and Movements." *American Journal of Physiology* 186:122-126, 1956.

15. RASCH, PHILIP J., and BURKE, ROGER K. *Kinesiology and Applied Anatomy*. Philadelphia: Lea & Febiger, 1967.

16. SLATER-HAMMEL, A. T. "Action Current Study of the Rectus Abdominalis As a Postural Muscle in Arm Movements." *Research Quarterly* 14:96, March, 1943.

17. WALLIS, EARL L., and LOGAN, GENE A. *Figure Improvement and Body Conditioning Through Exercise*. Englewood Cliffs: Prentice-Hall, Inc., 1964.

18. WORTZ, E. C., and PRESCOTT, E. J. "Effects of Subgravity Traction Simulation on the Energy Costs of Walking." *Aerospace Medicine* 37:1217-1222, December, 1966.

the serape effect

A serape is a brightly colored woolen blanket worn as an outer garment by people who live in Mexico or other Latin-American countries. A serape is designed to hang around the shoulders and cross diagonally on the anterior aspect of the trunk of the wearer. This is analogous to the direction of pull of a series of four pairs of muscles in the same general region covered by a serape. The four pairs of muscles are (1) rhomboids, (2) serratus anterior, (3) external obliques, and (4) internal obliques (Figures 9.1, 9.2, and 9.3). The serape effect is a synthesis of several major principles within analytic kinesiology designed to assist in the conceptualization of several interrelated aspects of anatomy and physics. (Logan and Wallis, 1960)

Muscular action by these four pairs of muscles working as a unit is called the *serape effect*. It is recognized that these muscles are assisted in the functions outlined below by the erector spinae and other muscles of the trunk. However, this discussion is limited to those muscles described as serape muscles. The serape effect incorporates several major concepts which are vital to an understanding of movement. In ballistic actions, such as throwing and kicking, the serape muscles add to the summation of internal forces. They also transfer internal force from a large body segment, the trunk, to relatively smaller body parts, the limbs. For example, the serape effect functions in throwing by summating, adding to, and transferring the internal forces generated in the lower limbs and pelvis to the throwing limb. *Summation of internal forces* is a major kinesiologic construct discussed in detail in Chapter 10.

The kinesiologic construct of summation of internal forces mentioned above must adhere to the Newtonian laws of motion. The reciprocal relationship between these laws and the serape effect can be observed during an analysis of throwing. A part of the body must first be set

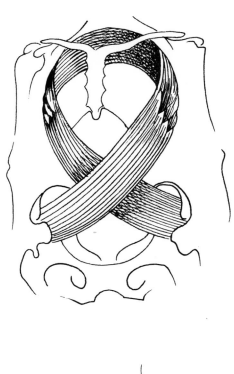

Figure 9.1. Serape—anterior view.

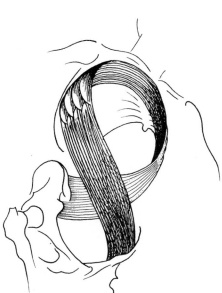

Figure 9.2. Serape—diagonal view.

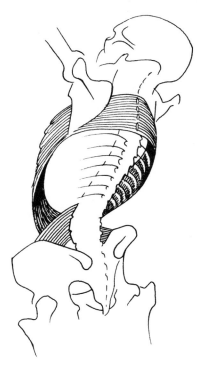

Figure 9.3. Serape—posterior view.

into motion in order that another segment will have something for the muscles to pull against to impart motion. When left transverse rotation of the pelvic girdle is initiated in the right-handed thrower, this is an application of Newton's Law of Inertia. Once the pelvis has been started in left transverse rotation, it will remain in motion unless acted upon by another force. This is an example of Newton's Law of Momentum. Concurrent with left transverse pelvic girdle rotation, the throwing limb is diagonally abducted and laterally rotated. This places three pairs of serape muscles on stretch. Prior to the time that the throwing arm is to be diagonally adducted and medially rotated, Newton's Third Law, The Law of Interaction, is operant. There is a definite interaction between the pelvic girdle on the left and the throwing limb on the right by way of concentric contraction of the left internal oblique, right external oblique, and serratus anterior on the right at the initiation of the throw. The pelvic girdle is rotating to the left, and the rib cage is rotating to the right.

Another component of the kinesiologic construct known as the summation of internal forces is observed during the serape effect. This is a phenomenon known as the *conservation of angular momentum.* Continuing with the throwing example, it can be observed that at the time the throwing limb is diagonally abducted and laterally rotated, the rib cage and pelvic girdle are at their farthest distance apart. This is seen at the point of maximum stretch by three pairs of serape muscles. At the initiation of medial rotation and diagonal adduction of the shoulder, diagonal flexion begins on the left side. This has the effect of shortening the radius of the long body lever. Shortening of this radius through flexion tends to increase the velocity of the moving body part. This internal force is transferred to the throwing limb in this example; consequently, the throwing limb's velocity is increased. This is an example of conservation of angular momentum.

The action of the internal and external obliques and serratus anterior performing their eccentric or lengthening action in preparation for the throw demonstrates a basic physiologic principle. *Muscles must be placed on their longest length in order to exert their greatest force.* As muscles decrease their length, their force decreases proportionally. Thus it can be seen that left transverse rotation of the pelvic girdle is absolutely essential for placing the serape muscles on stretch just prior to moving the throwing limb through the diagonal plane. This subtle rotary movement assists in placing these muscles on their maximum stretch.

In order to fully describe the serape effect, the functional relationship of the serape muscles on either side of the body must be considered. Starting with the rhomboids, which have a downward and lateral direction and attach proximally to the spinal column and distally to the vertebral border of the scapula, there is a functional completion of these muscles in the serratus anterior. The serratus anterior also attaches at the vertebral border of the scapula. The serratus anterior continues diagonally and downward as it attaches to the rib cage laterally and anteriorly. These two pairs of muscles work together on the vertebral border to move the scapula. Therefore, these serape muscles provide stability as well as movement of the scapula.

Continuing in a circular downward and diagonal direction on the rib cage is the external oblique on one side which continues into the internal oblique on the opposite side. The internal obliques terminate on the pelvis. When the bilateral pairs of these four muscles are considered, there are two diagonals crossing in front of the body working in conjunction with each other. This is a "muscular serape" wrapping diagonally around the trunk (Figure 9.4).

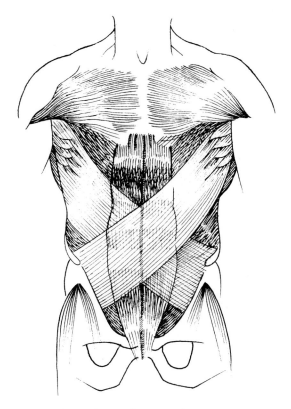

Figure 9.4. The muscular serape.

Critical analyses of forceful movement of the limbs indicate that most limb movements in sport tend to be diagonal in nature. One reason that movements are diagonal when one limb is used to impart force to an object is that the diagonally opposite limb is involved in maintaining balance when the performer is in the upright position. This is particularly true in such skills as throwing and kicking. Another reason that diagonal movements are the rule for most ballistic movements is that pendular levers revolving on multiaxis articulations tend to involve angular momentum, i. e., as an attempt is made to move a limb through a range of motion in one plane, there is a tendency for a lever or limb to describe a circle. Therefore, the limb moves in an arc diagonal to the long axis of the body because the joint involved is concurrently moving through space. Also, the spatial relationship of the musculature to the shoulder and hip joints indicates that a diagonal line of pull provides the most favorable arrangement for aggregate muscle action and the exertion of subsequent force.

There also appears to be some neurologic bases for diagonal movement patterns in man. One reflex adds some credibility to the diagonal movement pattern, the crossed-extensor reflex. Simply stated, this reflex is a combination of the flexion reflex in one limb and the extensor reflex occurring simultaneously in the opposite limb. This cross-extensor reflex is responsible for an "automatic relationship" in diagonal type movements. For example, the crossed-extensor reflex can be seen in the diagonal movement patterns of overarm pitching. When the right-handed pitcher starts his windup, there is an instant during the windup when his right elbow is almost fully extended and his left elbow is flexed. As movement continues toward the plate, the pitcher must conserve angular momentum within the throwing limb. To do this the right elbow is flexed, and at the same time, the left elbow is being extended—*throwing with force must involve both arms.* This constant reciprocal relationship between flexion and extension of alternate limbs, both upper and lower limbs, is commonly seen in many skills. Undoubtedly there are many other neurologic phenomena occurring during any diagonal-type movement. A discussion of these neurologic phenomena is beyond the scope and purpose of this book.

Dynamic stabilization is exemplified during the serape effect. (De-Mille, 1962) The dynamic stabilization function of the external and internal oblique muscles is probably most important for upper and lower limb movements. To continue with pitching skill as an example, one of the first basic movements for the right-handed pitcher is left transverse rotation of the pelvis. This means that the pelvic girdle must move counterclockwise to the longitudinal axis of his body. The left iliac crest is moving posteriorly as the right iliac crest is moving anteriorly. The muscles most involved for left transverse pelvic girdle rotation are the lateral and medial rotators of both hip joints. As the pelvis is moving in left transverse rotation, concentric contraction is occurring within the left external oblique and right internal oblique muscles. Concurrently, eccentric contraction is occurring within the right external oblique and left internal oblique muscles. This series of muscular contractions helps rotate the pelvis to the left side at the same time the rib cage is being rotated to the right side of the athlete. It can be seen that the left external oblique and right internal oblique muscles have been shortened as a unit. The right external oblique and left internal oblique muscles have been lengthened and placed on stretch as a unit. During these opposite rotations of the pelvic girdle and rib cage respectively, movement as well as relative stability has occurred between these two body segments. This is an example of *dynamic stabilization* (the Lomac Paradox). During this sequence of motion, preliminary forces have been established between the pelvic girdle and rib cage. The important serape muscles have been placed on stretch so subsequent force can be generated and movement can occur within the shoulder girdle, shoulder joint, and upper limbs.

To continue with the discussion of the serape effect as seen in throwing, the right upper limb of the right-handed thrower is diagonally abducted and laterally rotated during the preparatory phase. Concurrent with these movements, the scapula is being adducted by the rhomboids on the right side. In order for scapular adduction to occur, the serratus anterior muscle on the right side must contract eccentrically. Thus, three of the serape muscles are on stretch prior to the initial movement of the right upper limb in making the throw toward the plate. These three muscles of the serape must contract concentrically to transfer summated internal forces to the muscles most involved for diagonal adduction, medial rotation of the shoulder, and left diagonal flexion of the lumbar spine. While these three muscles within the serape are contracting concentrically to summate internal force for throwing, their three contralateral muscles are contracting eccentrically to provide dynamic stabilization.

The serape effect also plays a major role in forceful or ballistic movements of the lower limbs. When forceful movements of the lower limbs are seen, such as in punting or kicking, there is a reversal of the sequential movements of body segments. For example, during a forceful kick the serape muscles move the rib cage first. This is followed by movement within the pelvic girdle, which in turn adds to, summates, and transfers force to the kicking limb.

Many American football coaches teach their punters to move the kicking limb through an anteroposterior plane of motion. Although this concept is taught to some athletes, in reality the movement pattern of the kicking limb in the skilled punter is diagonal in nature (Figure 2.7). The reason for this lies in the fact that the spatial relationship of the muscles to the hip joint, particularly the adductors, will tend to pull the kicking lower limb through the diagonal plane of motion at the hip. Another factor contributing to this movement through a diagonal plane is the multiaxial arrangement of the hip joint. Since the soccer style of place-kicking more obviously employs movement through a diagonal plane of motion, it will be used as an example to explain the serape effect as it is related to transfer and summation of internal force to the lower limb. For sake of consistency, the kicking example will follow the same pattern as the discussion of throwing above.

A segment of the body must first be set into motion in order that another body segment will have something for muscles to pull against to impart motion. When the "right-legged" soccer-style place-kicker transfers his weight to the left lower limb or supportive limb, the left shoulder and left upper limb are diagonally abducted. Also, left diagonal extension is occurring in the lumbar spine. Concurrent with these motions, the rib cage is rotated to the left. This movement of the rib cage is allowed primarily by concentric contraction of the right external oblique and left internal oblique muscles. Their line of pull for this movement is from the right inferior aspect of the rib cage to the superior portion of the left side of the pelvic girdle. The left external oblique and right internal oblique are being placed on stretch, i. e., undergoing eccentric contraction. This, of course, is very important to the force generated within these muscles and ultimately summated and transferred to the kicking limb. As the rib cage is rotating to the left, right transverse pelvic girdle rotation is observed. This motion assists in the stretching or lengthening process within the left external oblique and right internal oblique muscles. Three serape muscles—the internal oblique on the right, external oblique on the left, and left serratus anterior—are all on stretch. Observation of the right hip joint of the kicker reveals that the kicking limb has been diagonally abducted and laterally rotated at this point. Lateral rotation is important because this places the muscles most involved on stretch for subsequent diagonal adduction and medial rotation. All of these motions can be considered as sequential, preparatory motions which summate, add to, and transfer force into the kicking limb. This force ultimately will be transferred to impart velocity to the ball.

To continue with the discussion of soccer-style place-kicking, a skill which requires a *continuous, sequential movement pattern* for greatest effectiveness, concentric contraction of the three serape muscles—the left serratus anterior, left external oblique, and right internal oblique—

causes left transverse rotation of the pelvic girdle. This results in right diagonal flexion of the lumbar spine, which tends to decrease the radius of the body as a lever. Thus, angular momentum is conserved and the velocity of the body segment involved is increased proportionately. All of these forces are sequentially transferred to the muscles most involved for diagonal adduction and medial rotation of the hip joint of the kicking limb. As the lower limb moves through the low diagonal plane of motion, the forces and momentum generated continue through the movement plane. The football or soccer ball is the recipient of these forces via the foot of the kicker.

The serape effect is a synthesis of a few major principles of analytic kinesiology designed to assist in the conceptualization of several interrelated aspects of anatomy and physics. The idea of the serape effect relates mainly to the function of the abdominal muscles when maximum force is desired in the use of the limbs. The purpose of presenting the serape effect is to provide the learner with a visual illustration indicating the function and importance of the interrelationship of pelvic girdle action when the upper and lower limbs are used. No new anatomic facts were introduced, but there was a new arrangement of known kinesiologic information. This concept is of value in teaching physical education skills, dance, and in the analysis of neuromuscular actions.

SELECTED REFERENCES

1. DeMille, Rosalind. Personal Correspondence, 1962.
2. Flint, M. M., and Gudgell, Janet. "Electromyographic Study of Abdominal Muscular Activity During Exercise." *Research Quarterly* 36:29-37, March, 1965.
3. Knott, Margaret, and Voss, Dorothy E. *Proprioceptive Neuromuscular Facilitation.* New York: Harper & Row, Publishers, 1968.
4. Logan, Gene A. "Movement in Art." *Quest* 2:42-45, April, 1964.
5. ———. *Adaptations of Muscular Activity.* Belmont: Wadsworth Publishing Co., Inc., 1964.
6. Logan, Gene A., and Wallis, Earl L. "Recent Findings in Learning and Performance." Southern Section Meeting, California Association for Health, Physical Education and Recreation, Pasadena City College, Pasadena, California (October, 1960).
7. Sheffield, Frederick J. "Electromyographic Study of the Abdominal Muscles in Walking and Other Movements." *American Journal of Physical Medicine* 41:142-147, August, 1962.

part three

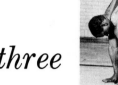

*kinesiologic
analysis*

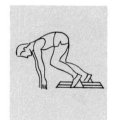

kinesiologic constructs

An understanding of human motion with respect to its application in sport, exercise, and dance requires knowledge of the interrelationships among myology, osteology, and some mechanical principles of physics. Two of the more important procedures used by the physical educator to improve neuromuscular skill are (1) application of knowledge of anatomic and mechanical principles of motion and (2) use of comparative noncinematographic and cinematographic analyses with the stereotype of "good form" for skill as seen during expert performances. The art of teaching results from successful transmission of knowledge in these areas to a lower-skilled performer who does not have the same physical and mental attributes of the expert performer. The real challenge of teaching is to assist performers to reach their skill potentials within their own anatomic, physiologic, and psychologic limitations. This is done best by the physical educator who expertly applies his knowledge of analytic kinesiology during the teaching-coaching process.

The physical educator must be able to communicate with the performer. The performer must be analyzed to determine major problems and he must be taught how to overcome those shortcomings in his performance. The effective teacher communicates to the performer only those pertinent facts which are necessary to increase the skill level. This is done by using a vocabulary understandable to the individual being taught. Therefore, the knowledgeable teacher must develop several vocabularies in order to impart information to students with varying backgrounds. The better physical educator acquires this knowledge and vocabularies through an intensive study of the scientific bases of physical education, sport theory, coaching methods, and through his own experiences as a performer.

A kinesiologic construct is a synthesis of kinesiologic subject matter derived primarily from anatomy and physics. There are three major

165

kinesiologic constructs: (1) summation of internal forces, (2) aerodynamic action of projectiles, and (3) hydrodynamics. The kinesiologic constructs within this chapter are oriented toward physics, but they have direct applications in regard to anatomy. The synthesis of kinesiologic subject matter within these constructs does not include any new facts. There is, however, a logical rearrangement of known facts.

Kinesiologic literature reveals a multitude of information related to human motion. A study of this voluminous information tends to inhibit the undergraduate student's "intellectual sight" to the point that it becomes difficult for him to "see the forest for the trees." Thus, the authors believe it is essential to synthesize this large amount of information related to kinesiology for the undergraduate student and present it in a non-mathematical framework. It is hoped that this will facilitate a better understanding of human motion and make this portion of kinesiology another "working tool" for the future physical educator as well as a progression into the study of biomechanics.

The undergirding bases upon which these three kinesiologic constructs were formed are the Newtonian Laws of Motion. These three kinesiologic constructs have been arranged and outlined to provide a better understanding of sequential human motion. They include the most pertinent facts and principles related to understanding and analyzing performance. *The understanding of analytic techniques and the ability to analyze are absolutely essential to be an effective physical educator.*

▶ Newtonian Laws of Motion

A working knowledge of Sir Isaac Newton's three laws of motion is essential in order to understand force (both internal and external forces) and its relationship to human movements. These laws were first stated by Newton during the seventeenth century. *Newton's laws involve inertia, acceleration, and reaction.*

The *Law of Inertia* is stated as follows: "Every body continues in a state of rest, or of uniform motion in a straight line, except and so far as it may be compelled by impressed forces to change that state." (Dyson, 1964) There are two concepts regarding inertia which must be understood. First, there is the concept of overcoming inertia when the body is at complete rest. This is the way one most readily conceptualizes forces and their action on a body at rest or inert. Second, inertia is also present when there is *uniform motion* in a straight line. To increase linear running speed, for example, additional internal force is required to overcome the type of inertia seen while the body is actually moving horizontally.

An example will help to clarify the Law of Inertia. The miler must overcome inertia in both ways. First, he must generate enough internal force to overcome external forces from the air and gravitational pull to start his inert body into motion. This is a more difficult process from the standpoint of energy expenditure than overcoming inertia once the body is moving. The miler in the example decides to run a three-minute fifty-five-second mile. In order to do this it was predetermined that it would take a fifty-nine-second pace on each of the first three 440-yard intervals. On the fourth 440-yard interval, inertia must be overcome again during the "kick phase" of the mile run. This is usually done within the last 110 yards of the race, i. e., the runner at that point in the mile run must volitionally call upon internal forces (muscular contractions) to change the state of *motion inertia*. This increases momentum during the "kick" and accelerates the body toward the finish line. This enables the runner to cover the final quarter mile in less than fifty-nine seconds; consequently, the time objective is attainable.

The *Law of Acceleration* is stated as follows: "The rate of change of momentum is proportional to the impressed force, and the actual change takes place in the direction the force acts." (Dyson, 1964)

To continue with the example of the miler, after inertia was overcome initially and pace established, momentum remained constant until the "kick" was started 110 yards from the finish line. With this set pace, forty-four seconds elapsed during the first 330 yards of the final 440 yards of the mile run. In order for the miler to run the planned mile in three minutes fifty-five seconds in this hypothetical example, pace must be increased to enable the miler to sprint the last 110 yards in fourteen seconds. In order to accomplish this, acceleration must occur. In this case, acceleration is a positive change in momentum. Since the Law of Acceleration states that the change in momentum is proportional to the impressed force, the miler must increase the internal force level by approximately one-third to cover the final 110 yards in fourteen seconds. Momentum was changed by directing the internally developed forces in a linear direction by pushing harder against the earth's surface while running with a forward body lean. A rate of change within the runner's momentum is also observed after crossing the finish line. Velocity at that time has a tendency to decrease sharply. This is an example of negative acceleration, or deceleration.

Momentum is the result of mass and velocity. Mass is the measure of an object's inertia. It is related to the resistance which an object will have to change in motion. Velocity is the distance an object travels during a known period of time.

The third law of motion is the *Law of Reaction*. It is stated as follows: "To every action there is an equal and opposite reaction; or the mutual actions of two bodies in contact are always equal and opposite in direction." (Dyson, 1964) The adherence to this law can be seen in the example of the miler. As he is running forward with a slight body lean, there is a diagonal force exerted backward against the surface of the earth. This "action force" is the direct result of the summation of internal forces. Gravitational force also causes the body to exert force against the earth. The "reaction force" is the surface of the earth pushing back toward the mass of the runner. Because of the differences in size of these two objects, the miler and earth, it is obvious that there will be no visible reaction of the earth. Therefore, owing to this type of reaction on the part of the earth, the linear motion reaction of the miler is enhanced.

Another example of the Law of Reaction can be seen in platform diving. When a diver executes a twisting dive *while in the air*, i. e., rotational movement occurs around the longitudinal axis of the body, there will be marked action with an opposite reaction. When the upper limbs are moved clockwise around the longitudinal axis of the body (action), the body itself will move counterclockwise around its longitudinal axis (reaction). On the other hand, if the diver initiates a twisting dive *before leaving the platform*, the twist will be in the direction of the initial upper limb movement. This, at first observation, seems to be a contradiction of the Law of Reaction. However, there is a similarity between this example and the one given for the miler. The diver in this example initiates an action and the reaction is not observed because the force is exerted against a heavy platform attached to the surface of the earth. Owing to the obvious differences in size between these objects and the diver, the reaction occurs in the subsequent performance of the athlete.

▶ Summation of Internal Forces

The kinesiologic construct of summation of internal forces is presented herein as a three-part model. To perform a sport skill, there are usually three general phases through which the performer must move sequentially. These are classified as (1) the preparation phase, (2) the movement phase, and (3) the follow-through and/or recovery phase. In addition, a preliminary stance must also be considered for many skills. Summation of internal force is seen primarily throughout the completion of the first two sequential phases. The follow-through and/or recovery phase as discussed is a deceleration of forces, but it is an integral part of the overall skill. Owing to rules limitations and the nature of many sport skills, the performer must recover to be able to make subsequent movement, avoid injury, and prepare to summate forces to execute the next movement or skill. The concepts discussed below in the model do not apply in all cases to all sports skill. *This sequential*

*model is meant to be a guide for observing a performer from the start
to the completion of movement.*

PREPARATION PHASE—The preparation phase is important because
the quality of movement leading into the preparation portion of the skill
will have either a beneficial or detrimental effect upon subsequent movement. The demands of each sport skill dictate the type of preparation
necessary for subsequent movement. In some sport skills, the athlete
must move rapidly from a stance, and in other skills some stability is
necessary to receive an external force. A proper preparation phase is
often overlooked during teaching and analytic processes. For example,
when an athlete assumes a stance, if the muscles most involved in the
performance to summate internal forces are not on their greatest length,
the ultimate summation of forces will not be of an appreciable magni-
tude. *The force exerted by a muscle is porportional to its length.* (*Muscle
length-force ratio*[1]) Although a muscle group responds with its greatest
force when placed on its greatest length, it is not always desirable to
apply this directly to some sport skills. Many times other factors such
as direction of subsequent movement and equilibrium are involved, and
these factors might contraindicate the use of maximum internal force.

*In sport skills requiring considerable stability or equilibrium, the
center of gravity of the body must be lowered.* (*Stable base of support*)
In the bipedal stance, this is done mainly by flexion at the knee and
hip joints. Offensive, interior football linemen utilize this principle when
forming a protective "passing pocket" for the quarterback. Each pass-
protection blocker must use a wide base of support for stability. This
is absolutely necessary to maintain the upright position when hitting
and being hit by the defensive linemen. Also, from this stable position
centers, guards, and tackles are capable of moving in any direction required depending on the situation.

The exact center of gravity of the body must be assumed. There
are detailed scientific procedures for determining the body's center of
gravity, but these are not of prime importance to the general application
of kinesiologic analyses on a day-to-day basis. The center of gravity
of the total body should be considered only as a general reference point
because, as an example, it can lie outside of the body during high-
jumping. As a general rule, however, the center of gravity is in the
middle of the pelvic girdle when the individual is in the upright position.

Many skills require the body to be in a state of equilibrium part
time or at all times during the execution of the performance. *This state*

---

1. The term "muscle length-force ratio" is used as a recall phrase. This and
subsequent phrases are indicated for each mechanical principle used during analytic
procedures, see Figure 12.2.

*of equilibrium is accomplished when the center of gravity lies within
the body's base of support.* (*Maintenance of body equilibrium*) If the
center of gravity falls outside its base of support, movement will occur
in the direction in which equilibrium was lost. This is commonly observed in the processes of walking and running because both of these
skills involve a series of alternately losing and regaining equilibrium.
During a relatively fast start, the center of gravity should be high. It
should also be as near as possible to the edge of the base of support
in the stance before the start is begun. Good track starting techniques
for the sprinter take full advantage of this principle. The sprinter's hands
are his primary base of support, and the center of gravity is relatively
high during the stance and preparatory phases. As soon as there is movement of the hands upward from the track at the sound of the gun, the
sprinter must propel himself forward into the movement phase or fall
(Figure 10.1).

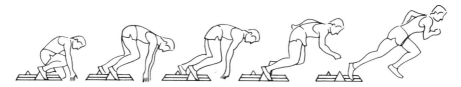

Figure 10.1.   Losing and controlling equilibrium.

MOVEMENT PHASE—The main purpose of the preparation phase was
to prepare the individual for the effort to summate internal forces needed
to perform a skill. Internal forces are actually summated during the
movement phase. The unique nature of each skill predetermines the
specific sequence of joint actions for the summation of internal forces.
The amount of force required is specifically dependent upon the skill
to be performed. According to Gardner, "only as much speed or force
as a situation demands should be used. Great speed or force makes control more difficult." (Gardner, 1963) Regardless of the amount of force
required, every skill requires a timed and sequential summation of internal forces. It is obvious, as examples, that the force required in shuffle-
board skill is not as great as that required to put the sixteen-pound shot.
However, in both instances, there is a definite necessity for timed and
sequential summation of internal forces to perform in a skilled manner.
    *Summation of internal forces is a direct result of a rapid, timed
sequence of aggregate muscle actions moving body parts in such a way
that each force is added to the preceding force to provide the desired*

amount of force at the specific point of application. (Kinetic chain) For example, internal force is summated for throwing by sequential and timed aggregate muscle contractions occurring at the ankle, knee, hip, pelvic girdle, spinal column, shoulder, elbow, radio-ulnar, wrist, and inter-phalangeal joints. Thus, it can be seen that the resultant force, which began at the ankle joint or feet, was ultimately transferred to the object to be thrown (Figure 10.2).

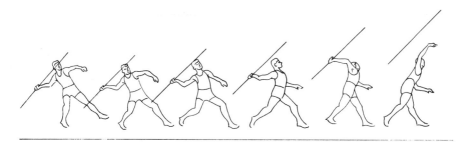

Figure 10.2. Kinetic chain as seen in javelin throwing.

When summating internal forces, the speed of each body part being moved should exceed the velocity of the preceding body part. (Pro-gressive, sequential segment velocity) For greatest efficiency of move-ment or performance, the mass of the contracting musculature must be taken into consideration. Smaller muscle groups tend to contract faster than larger muscle groups. Therefore, *the transfer of force from one body segment to another should be from larger or stronger muscle groups to smaller or weaker muscle groups. (Large to small muscle force transfer)*

In all skills force for the movement of the body mass should be applied as nearly as possible in the direction of the intended motion. (Force application in intended direction) This is necessary to allow as much force as possible to be utilized at the completion of the summation of internal forces. If this is done, there will be a relatively small amount of force dissipated. An example of how this principle is utilized in sport is seen in American football blocking. It is essential that the offensive lineman apply force directly toward the center of the mass of his op-ponent because football rules dictate that hands cannot be used in the process of blocking. If the offensive lineman makes contact in the center of his opponent's mass (midsection), he can move his opponent in any desired direction by utilizing the summation of internal forces starting with plantar flexion at the ankle. If, on the other hand, he does not make blocking contact within the opponent's center of mass, application of forces will be ineffective and the opponent will tend to rotate from the ineffective force and from the block. By applying force in a direction away from the intended motion, some of the force developed on the part of the offensive lineman in making his block is wasted or dissipated. Such an offensive blocker would soon find himself sitting next to the coach on the bench.

When imparting force to external objects or propelling the body when horizontal distance is of prime importance, the greatest speed possible should be attained at the moment of projection. (*Projection speed*) Obtaining maximum horizontal distance is of importance in such events as shot-putting, long-jumping, triple-jumping, long shots in basketball, and home run-hitting in baseball. For the execution of these skills, and others, *there is always timed sequence of movement involving an interrelationship between linear and angular motions.* (*Combined linear-angular motions*) It can be seen in Figure 10.2 that javelin-throwing involves both linear and angular motions. The mass of the body is moving linearly through space as a result of the angular motion taking place within the joints of the lower limbs. When linear motion has been established at a constant rate of speed, the javelin thrower must go through a series of complicated cross-over steps to integrate this linear motion with further angular motions to produce a series of angular motions resulting in a terminal diagonal movement of the upper throwing limb. Javelin-throwing is one of the most complicated field events because of the difficulty of efficiently integrating linear motion with angular motion.

Shortening the radius of a limb or body part will increase the speed at the moving end of the limb or body part. (*Conservation of angular momentum*) Shortening the radius of motion results in an increase of angular velocity within the moving limb or body part. This type of increase in angular velocity is seen very commonly in sport skills. This concept of motion is important because it facilitates the integration of linear and angular motions. It also helps in the timing of motion between body parts. It was stated above that the speed of each body part should be faster than that of the preceding body part. The increase in angular velocity in a throwing limb, for example, adds more potential force which can add greater velocity to the thrown ball. *Conversely, lengthening a limb or body part will have a tendency to reduce angular velocity within the limb or body part involved.* (*Limb or segment deceleration*)

These procedures of increasing and decreasing angular velocity are commonly observed when watching a rebound tumbler in action. If the rebound tumbler performs a front flip rapidly while in the air above the trampoline bed, it is best performed in a full tuck position. In other words, the performer "bunches the body" by extreme flexion at the knee, hip, and lumbar spine joints. This shortens the body as a lever toward its center of gravity. The body is turning around its center of gravity in space. The body must increase in speed to cover the same amount of distance it would cover through the larger arc if the body were in a full lay-out or full lever position. The skilled rebound tumbler can move from the tight tuck position to the lay-out position. This is done primarily to slow the rate of rotation around the body's center of gravity. This is often done to move the body into position for a subsequent full body drop as well as to reduce the body's angular velocity.

The weight of the sport implement or object to be thrown must be taken into consideration. *If the object is relatively heavy in relation to the size and strength of the individual, one or both feet must be kept in contact with the ground at the moment the implement is projected from the limb into the air.* (*Foot contact at projection*) (Figure 10.3)

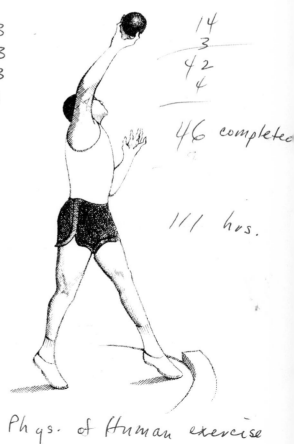

Figure 10.3. Foot contact at moment of shot projection.

One immediately thinks of the sixteen-pound shot put when considering this concept; however, other commonly used sport implements might well be considered to be heavy objects. For example, there would be some sixth-grade boys and girls who would find the twelve-inch softball to be a heavy object when it is thrown for distance during a skill test. The size and strength of an individual in relation to the weight of the object to be thrown must be evaluated by the physical educator.

The position of the feet on the ground at the time of release is very important, because if the feet leave the ground prior to release of the sport implement or ball, the summation of internal forces will be interrupted and force will be dissipated. Also, the foot or feet remaining in contact with the ground tend to insure that the force will be imparted in the desired direction.

Other factors must be considered when handling relatively light objects in a variety of sports. If the object is light compared with the performer's strength and other anatomic features, the feet might well be completely off the floor when the object is released, or one foot might be on the playing surface when the object is released. Such factors as velocity, accuracy, and strategy must be taken into consideration when applying this principle. For example, the baseball pitcher is dealing with a relatively light object, the regulation baseball, during the pitching process. If the pitcher threw the baseball toward the batter with both feet on the ground, his summation of internal forces would be impeded and the hitter would take full advantage of this weakness. At the time the baseball is released, the left foot of the right-handed pitcher is in contact with the ground. The basketball player executing the jump shot releases the ball when both feet are off the court. This is done, of course, to gain a height advantage over the opponent. The summation of internal forces required in these examples is not as great as the summation of internal forces required to put the sixteen-pound shot. The volleyball spiker spikes the ball while both feet are off the court. This is done to gain an angle and height advantage over the opposition. The volleyball spike may be imparted with great force or relatively light force; thus, strategy is also involved in this skill.

There are many sports where athletes must use implements such as bats, hockey sticks, and rackets. When implements are used, it is imperative that the grip be maintained firmly prior to and at the point of impact to transfer the summation of internal forces effectively to the implement and subsequently to the object to be struck. (Grip) If the grip is not maintained through the point of impact, force will be partially dissipated. Several products, such as rosin, pine tar, golf gloves, and other commercial products, are placed on the hands by athletes to insure firm grips.

FOLLOW-THROUGH AND RECOVERY PHASES—The follow-through and recovery phases of a skill involve slowing, stopping, and recovery of the body or its parts to make subsequent movements demanded of the performer. The nature of the sport or activity, rules of the sport, and strategy used by the athlete will determine how he acts or reacts during the follow-through and/or recovery phase. It can easily be observed that the rules and the nature of the sport often have a direct bearing on the execution of the sport skill. As examples, the baseball pitcher and javelin thrower are both interested in imparting the greatest amount of force possible to their respective sport objects, the ball and javelin. The baseball pitcher is not only interested in velocity, but he also must be concerned more with accuracy than the javelin thrower. Rules for baseball-pitching are more stringent than the rules for javelin-throwing. In addition, the baseball pitcher must be ready to field a hit ball immediately after he pitches. He must also be concerned with his own self-protection. This places some unusual demands upon his recovery after throwing the ball toward the plate. On the other hand, the javelin thrower need only avoid crossing the fault line during his follow-through or recovery phase. He can literally propel himself through the air and land on his abdomen if he desires because he knows that his sport obligation has finished with his follow-through phase. Someone else will retrieve his javelin and return it to him. The baseball batter does not have the same obligation regarding the return of the baseball to the pitcher.

Virtually all sport skills have a follow-through or recovery phase. Therefore, the physical educator must concern himself with the best principles of motion related to the limitations imposed upon the performer by the rules of the game.

The extent of the follow-through is in direct proportion to the intensity of the summation of internal forces. (Follow-through intensity) A follow-through should be smooth and continuous in order to dissipate the amount of force accumulated during the summation of internal forces. It is necessary to stop the body and its limbs and to prepare for subsequent motion. If the follow-through tends to be "jerky" or stops too soon, this may be a result of inadvertently slowing the summation of internal forces prior to the crucial phase of the sport skill. The physical educator should analyze the follow-through as a special phase of the sport skill in order to gain some insight into the effectiveness of the performer's summation of internal forces.

Most sports require a series of integrated skills which are performed sequentially. This series of sport skills requires the performer to accelerate and decelerate his internal forces. In many situations the athlete never has the opportunity to fully recover prior to moving to the next objective within the contest. As a result, the athlete, like the chess player, must think of his "moves" in advance. During the recovery phase, the athlete may be confronted with a number of alternatives: (1) bringing his body to a complete stop (deceleration), (2) changing the total direction of the body, or (3) overcoming inertia while in motion (acceleration). *When stopping quickly, changing direction, or receiving force, the base of support should be widened in order to lower the center of gravity. (Directional change)*

Examples of stopping and changing direction are commonly observed in a soccer game. There are times when a soccer player must sprint at full speed for several yards in order to position himself to "head" a soccer ball. As the spot is approached where the soccer ball is to be hit with the head, it may be necessary to come to a complete stop. To do this the soccer player simply widens his base of support. This is accomplished by abducting both lower limbs at the hip joint. The soccer player widens his base of support and lowers his center of gravity in this example. There are at least three reasons for this action: (1) to stop his linear motion, (2) to maintain his equilibrium, or (3) to place his extensor muscle groups on stretch. The latter is necessary to reinitiate summation of internal forces to "head the soccer ball." The skilled soccer player must be able to kick the soccer ball while running at full speed and continue his run in pursuit of the ball following the kick. This skill demands that he maintain his equilibrium at all times. This is done by the soccer player widening his base of support, resulting in a lower center of gravity by means of hip and knee flexions. After he kicks the ball, he must consider his next alternative.

The rebound tumbler utilizes these techniques of motion in order to stop vertical motion after a rebound tumbling routine. In order for the gymnast to stop himself at the conclusion of a rebound tumbling skill, flexion must occur at the ankle, knee, and hip joints as contact is made with the bed. Also, the base of support must be widened to maintain stability. By doing these two basic maneuvers, the gymnast brings himself to a stop. Therefore, the performer has controlled his own force as well as the force generated by the movement of the trampoline bed. The rebound tumbler has absorbed the external forces from the movement of the trampoline bed as well as dissipating his own internal forces to bring himself to a complete stop.

Some sport skills require the athlete to absorb shock derived from the force of the event during the recovery phase of the skill. *In sport skills where it is necessary to absorb shock derived from internal as well as external forces, force should be dissipated over as large a surface area as possible. (Force dissipation)* As examples, the pole vaulter and high jumper must be concerned with utilizing this principle of motion during the recovery phase of their events. It is not uncommon for a good pole vaulter to fall fifteen or sixteen feet through space during his follow-through or recovery phase. The vaulter must land in a position in the pit to dissipate force so he will not injure himself. This is done by exposing a large portion of the back to the receiving surface. The high jumper uses the same technique with the addition of rolling and spreading the force over a large area. The shoulder roll used very commonly by foot-ball players after they are hit is another example of how force can be dissipated over a large portion of the athlete's body, thus tending to reduce injury. The sport of judo incorporates falling techniques to absorb shock. This is done by exposing large surfaces of the body to the mat and by preliminary slapping with the forearm and outstretched hand (Figure 10.4). An accompanying yell allows maximum exhalation of air.

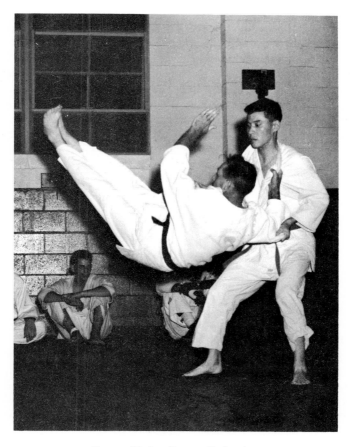

Figure 10.4. Force dissipation.

► **Aerodynamics**

As a kinesiologic construct, *aerodynamics* deals with the flight of objects acted upon by air resistance and gravity. It must be remembered that the human body is often an airborne object as it performs many skills. Consequently, it must conform in these situations to the laws of aerodynamics.

During the movement phase of the summation of internal forces, the power was generated to transfer the internal force from the body to propel the body itself into the air or to propel another object into the air. Consequently, aerodynamics comes into play at the time the object becomes airborne as a result of the summation of internal forces. *Aerodynamics is concerned with the angle of projection, flight pattern of the projectile, the object in flight, and the reaction of the object when it strikes a surface.*

Such events as the triple jump and diving are examples of the human body used as a projectile at the conclusion of the summation of internal forces. The discus- and hammer-throwing events in track and field are examples of events where a sport implement becomes the projectile.

Sport implements are used by athletes as extensions of their bodies to add leverage and force to the object propelled into the air. Some sport implements are used for throwing purposes and others are used for hitting purposes. Examples of sport implements used for throwing purposes are found in lacrosse and jai alai. The tennis racket and baseball bat are examples of sport implements used for hitting or striking purposes.

ANGLE OF PROJECTION—*The optimum angle of projection for an object is dependent upon the nature or physical characteristics of the object as well as the objectives of the skill. (Angle of projection)* It is obvious that the air resistance quotients of the human body, shot put, discus, or javelin are considerably different. Another physical consideration is the actual weight of an object. The factors of distance and accuracy must also be considered when determining the optimum angle of projection for any performance.

Theoretically, the optimum angle for the projection of an object is forty-five degrees. However, observations of athletes performing skills requiring objects to be propelled through space indicate that angles of less than forty-five degrees are generally seen. This is particularly true when the human body is the object to be propelled of its own initiative through space. The difficulty lies in the problem of integrating linear velocity with angular velocity at the moment of take-off. This phenomenon is observed in the long jump. Linear momentum is decreased at the moment of take-off if the take-off angle is increased. The reason for this lies in the fact that the antigravity muscles must work against the pull of gravity in lifting the body vertically. If linear velocity is lost, the body will not travel as far horizontally through space at the higher take-off angle. This, of course, would ultimately decrease the distance traversed by the long jumper. The object in long-jumping is to jump as far as possible. Consequently, most long jumpers will have a take-off angle considerably less than forty-five degrees. The take-off angle is usually found in the thirty-degree range. The shot-putter's angle of projection would be nearer forty-five degrees. There are many other factors to be taken into consideration such as length of the jumper's lower limbs, linear velocity at the time of take-off, strength of extensor or antigravity muscles, length of the approach, air density, altitude, and body weight.

▶ Flight Pattern

The angle of projection determines the path through which the object will move while in the air. This flight path is known as a *parabola*. The reference point for describing the parabolic flight pattern of an object is its center of gravity. *Once the object is airborne, no movement by the object around its center of gravity will change the trajectory or parabolic flight pattern. (Parabola)* (Figure 10.5). Gravity and air resistance as

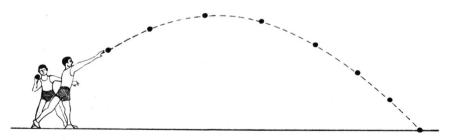

Figure 10.5. Parabola of a shot.

external forces do have an effect upon projected objects. The effect of gravity is a constant in performances, and air resistance is a variable factor. Movements made while in the air by tumblers, divers, long jumpers, and high jumpers, as examples, will not alter the parabolic flight pattern of their centers of gravity. Many believe erroneously that the extra movement of limbs on the part of the long jumper while he is in the mid-air position during his parabolic flight pattern will increase the horizontal distance of the long jump. In reality, this series of extra-

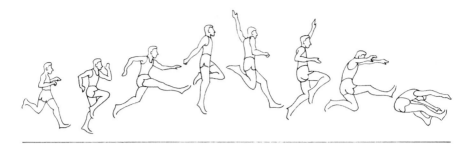

Figure 10.6. Efficient limb action in flight.

neous motions is a waste of energy and is more likely to have an adverse effect upon horizontal distance than a beneficial effect upon it. Figure 10.6 shows a long jumper who uses a minimum amount of limb movement in flight.

THE OBJECT IN FLIGHT—An object in flight is directly affected by the external forces of air resistance and gravity. Air resistance is considered herein since it is a variable entity. The flight of the object will be affected by the extent of air movement. When the air is calm, it is relatively easy to predict the flight pattern of a projected object. However, it is rare to have a completely calm atmosphere when participating in an athletic event outdoors. The direction, velocity, and variability of the wind must be considered as external factors which may have a bearing on the flight pattern of the object. These factors have a direct bearing many times on athletic strategy. For example, the tennis player must make adjustments each time he changes courts to allow for the direction and gustiness of the wind.

The main factors to be considered while a sport object is in flight are (1) *the velocity of the object at the time it becomes airborne (flight velocity)*, (2) *density of the air through which the object is flying (air density)*, (3) *shape of the object (sport object's shape)*, (4) *angle of the object in flight (flight angle)*, (5) *area of the object's surface (surface area)*, (6) *texture of the surface area (texture-friction factor)*, and (7) *rotation of the object while in flight (spin)*.

The momentum imparted to the object at release is directly proportional to the summation of internal forces. The greater the velocity of the object, the greater the horizontal distance covered while in flight. This is dependent upon the angle of projection and resultant parabola as well as the effect of air resistance. There are optimum and specific velocities for each sport skill. For the athlete who is trying to cover a maximum horizontal distance with his own body, his flight speed through the parabola must be as great as he can possibly attain. On the other hand, when accuracy is of prime importance, the flight speed of the sport object may never reach its maximum. As an example, many basketball passes involve a submaximal flight speed because greater velocities would adversely affect accuracy and ball-handling.

Air temperature, humidity, barometric pressure, and altitude have a bearing on air density. The physical educator must be concerned with one or all of these factors when working with athletes who will propel objects into the air. For example, due to differences in altitude, the air is less dense in Mexico City, Mexico, than in Long Beach, California. A 160-pound long jumper capable of running a 9.5 second 100-yard dash will jump approximately three inches farther in Mexico City than in Long Beach, California.

Sport objects propelled through the air have a wide variety of shapes. Some of these lend themselves very effectively to flight. Others are designed very inefficiently for maximum flight. The human body is a good example of the latter, and the javelin is a good example of the former. Each sport object responds in a specific way to air resistance. As examples, the football, discus, and javelin all gain horizontal distance by being thrown into a head wind provided that the head wind velocity is not great enough to negate linear motion. On the other hand, spheroid objects such as baseballs and softballs are adversely affected by any head wind in terms of their horizontal distance and flight velocity. Generally, the more "streamlined" the human body becomes during flight, the less air resistance will play an adverse role during the performance. Even the stability of a streamlined object such as a javelin and football must be maintained during flight to limit the adverse effects of air resistance. This is done by projecting these objects into their flight patterns with sufficient amount of rotation around their longitudinal axes to maintain stability in flight.

The shape of the object has a direct bearing on the airflow past its surfaces, and this is a factor which affects flight due to differences in air resistances on the surfaces. For example, the spinning discus must be projected similar to an aircraft wing on takeoff to obtain maximum advantage of lift from the air. This position allows the discus to obtain an optimum lift due to negative pressure on its upper surface and positive or lifting pressure on its lower surface. The discus will tend to "stall" if it is projected in a position too vertical to the earth. If it is projected horizontal to the earth, its position and shape does not lend itself to added lift from airflow. The horizontal distance obtained in this case will be primarily due to the athlete's summation of internal forces without the advantage of any subsequent lift by the air. The commonly observed "curve phenomenon" by projected spheroid sport objects is directly due to spin direction, air resistance, gravitational effects, and uneven airflow around the spinning object while it is in flight. Figure 10.7 illustrates airflow, spin direction, and air turbulence of pitched baseballs thrown as curves, fast balls, and knucklers.

The larger the total surface area of the sport object, the greater the potential reaction to air resistance and wind resistance. For example, a baseball and regulation softball are nearly comparable in weight. The twelve-inch softball, however, has a greater surface area to respond to air resistance; consequently, the softball pitcher can cause a greater curve through a shorter distance than a baseball pitcher.

The physical weight of a sport object will have a direct bearing on its flight pattern and movements in flight. An obvious example of this is a comparison of flight patterns of a golf ball and a table tennis ball. Both of these spheroid objects have approximately the same amount of surface area; however, they differ appreciably in regard to weight. If hit with maximum force into a crosswind, the heavier golf ball will travel over a much greater horizontal distance. The lighter table tennis ball's horizontal distance will be adversely affected by the effects of the crosswind because of its light weight.

The texture (smoothness or roughness) of the surface of the sport object will have a direct bearing on the object in flight. The rougher the surface area of a sport object, the greater the amount of friction created between the object in flight and the air. The greater the friction factor, the greater potential for spin up to a point. The condition of a sport object's surface may well change during the course of the athletic contest. For example, as the new tennis ball becomes worn, it loses the amount of friction it can create against the air. This will cause a change

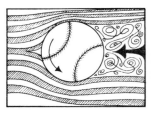 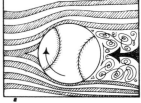 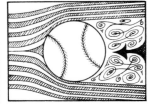

Curve Ball—Forward and diagonal rotation causes accelerated air streamlines on top of the ball which force it downward.

Fast Ball—Backward rotation causes increased velocities in air streamlines under the ball; consequently, the ball will rise if thrown with great velocity.

Knuckle Ball—Lack of rotation and interaction with turbulence area immediately behind the ball causes an erratic flight pattern.

Figure 10.7. Aerodynamics of pitched balls.

in the flight pattern of the tennis ball when it is struck and when it rebounds from the court. A change in surface area texture is also seen at times in baseball games. A baseball is relatively smooth, but the seams serve as a rough portion of the ball to create friction while the ball is in flight. The "spit ball" or "Vaseline ball" thrown by some pitchers produces an ultrasmooth surface on the baseball. This contrasts sharply with the rough seam area. This variation in surfaces on the baseball causes an erratic flight pattern. A wet surface area causes the surface of a sport object to become smoother, thus decreasing the amount of friction between the ball and the air. This creates erratic flight patterns due to loss of stability in flight.

The primary effect of rotation of an object in flight is to add stability. Rotation of a sport object is called "spin." A ball or thrown object will tend to curve in the direction of its spin. A baseball pitcher throws the fast ball by using back-spin. (Back-spin means that the top of the ball is rotating back toward the pitcher.) This back-spin provides a greater lift on the ball *if* it is thrown with great velocity because the air flows past the ball's upper and lower surfaces, and the airflow tends to be faster on the bottom portion of the ball than on the upper surface. This brings about a pressure difference which causes the ball to rise when thrown with great velocity by a skilled pitcher. The average pitcher's fast ball will not rise when it covers the sixty feet six inches because it is not thrown with spin and velocity great enough to counteract the pull of gravity. Consequently, the average fast ball appears to be straight. Conversely, forward rotation of a ball in flight will cause it to drop toward earth faster than gravity in the direction of its spin. "Pure forward rotation" is not commonly observed in pitched baseballs because of the release difficulties involving the elbow, radio-ulnar, and wrist joints.

A ball can also be thrown or hit to make it curve left or right. This is done by striking the ball on its left or right surface. Thus there is created a sideward and forward spin causing the ball to curve in the direction of the spin. Spin, therefore, increases the stability and predictability of the flight pattern of the sport object when it is put into flight by a skilled athlete. On the other hand, when a sport object is put into flight without spin even by a skilled athlete, the object will lack stability, and the flight path of the object will not be predictable. The nonrotating sport object will have a very erratic flight pattern due to an imbalance of pressure forces exerted at the side and rear of the sport object as it encounters varying pressure levels during its flight. Even the expert knuckle-ball pitcher does not know at the time of release whether the ball will traverse the strike zone, hit the batter, or bounce in front of the plate.

REACTION OF THE OBJECT WHEN IT STRIKES A SURFACE—A knowledge of rebounding objects is essential because there are many times in sport when the performer must deal with a rebounding sport object in a variety of ways. In many sports the ability to win the contest is actually dependent upon the skill of the athlete to handle rebounds effectively. As examples, the handling of rebounds is essential in such sports as tennis, handball, basketball, ice hockey, squash rackets, jai alai, table tennis, and fielding in baseball and soft ball. Rebound will be affected by at least five factors: (1) the angle of the sport object's approach to the striking surface, (2) rotation or spin of the sport object when it hits or rebounds against the striking surface, (3) composition or texture of the striking surface, (4) composition (texture and elasticity) of the sport object, and (5) the contour or shape of the surface which is struck.

Generally, the angle of a sport object's rebound is similar to its angle of approach to the surface to be struck. (Angle of incidence) The actual rebound angle is directly affected by the factors mentioned above, as well as by gravitational forces and air resistance.

The angle of rebound from the surface by the sport object will be dependent upon the direction of rotation or spin of the sport object when it strikes the surface. (Angle of rebound) A ball or sport object without spin tends to rebound near the same angle as its approach angle. *On the other hand, a spinning sport object will tend to rebound in the direction of its spin.* For the most part, athletes deal with rebounding objects from vertical and horizontal surfaces. As an example, the basketball backboard is a vertical surface which must be dealt with during a basketball game. Some basketball players utilize the backboard when shooting free throws. When the ball is shot with considerable backspin, this causes the ball to drop toward the basket after it has rebounded from the backboard. Tennis players must deal with rebounds from a horizontal surface. The right-handed tennis player will oftentimes serve by imparting spin to the ball by hitting it on its right side causing it to spin diagonally around its vertical axis. When it rebounds from the opposite court, it will reflect from the court in the direction of its spin. Varying the velocity and spin of a ball is another important strategic aspect of many sports.

The composition of the striking surface will have an effect on the rebound of the sport object. Friction and resiliency of the struck surface are both important considerations. (*Surface friction and resiliency*) Atmospheric conditions will also have a direct bearing on outdoor surfaces in regard to their friction and resiliency aspects. The condition of outdoor surfaces will vary during any twenty-four-hour period depending upon the amount of moisture in the air. Artificial turf is not as adversely affected by weather conditions; consequently, rebounds of sport objects from artificial turf tend to be more consistent than rebounds of the same sport objects on outdoor or natural turfs.

The degree of elasticity or "give" has a direct bearing upon the angle of rebound of a sport object. (*Elasticity*) Elasticity is the ability of a sport object to return to its original shape after it has been struck or has struck a surface. Some sport objects when struck compress to as much as one-half their original size. Thus, it is important to have balls of consistent elasticity in a contest. For example, increased elasticity due to the age of a tennis ball can distort timing because the ball will compress more when hit and remain on the racket a fraction of a second longer. Where a ball with less elasticity would clear the net, the ball with increased elasticity is more likely to be hit into the net. The texture of the outer surface of the sport object will also have an effect on the rebound angle as well as the texture which is to be struck.

The contour or shape of the striking surface influences the rebound. (*Striking surface shape*) A variety of striking surfaces are seen in sport. Catgut or nylon strings of a tennis racket, curvilinear or cupped hand of the handball player, round surface of the baseball bat, flat surface of the hockey stick, strings of the lacrosse stick, and irregular surface of the shoes worn by kickers in soccer and American football are a few examples. Controlling the rebound angle of a sport object is largely dependent upon the nature and shape of the striking surface. For example, some people have indicated that the most difficult skill in all of sport is hitting a baseball since the athlete is trying to strike a spheroid object (ball) with a cylindrical object (bat). This is especially difficult because two convex surface areas do not allow for a large hitting surface, and this leaves very little margin for error. Soccer-style place-kicking in American football is more accurate than traditional place-kicking techniques. The reasons for this are (1) the ball is struck by a greater surface area allowing better control and (2) the diagonal adduction movement of the lower limb involves a larger muscle mass and a more natural movement. *Generally, the more surface area exposed at the time the sport object is struck, the greater potential control by the athlete over the rebound angle of the sport object.* (*Rebound surface area*)

▶ **Hydrodynamics**

A basic understanding of the kinesiologic construct of hydrodynamics is of vital importance because the physical educator is often called upon to teach a wide variety of swimming skills.

The main difference between movement in the water as opposed to movement on land is the difference in gravitational pull. The effects of gravity are relatively negated when a body is fully or partially submerged in water. Buoyancy is the primary concern when in water. Buoyancy is the upward pressure exerted by the water in which the body is emersed. (*Buoyancy*) If the weight of the water displaced is greater than that of the body, the body is lifted to the surface. If the weight of the water displaced is less than that of the body, the body will sink. It is a well-known fact that some people have better buoyancy than others. This is due primarily to the fact that there is disparity between individuals in regard to the ratio of body fat to bone and muscle. The individual with a greater amount of body fat tends to be more buoyant. This is one reason that the well-conditioned athlete with a low body fat ratio will tend to be a "sinker." This is also the reason why most women tend to be buoyant, because their ratio of fat to bone and muscle is greater than men's.

Propulsive force in the water is usually preceded by a propulsive force from land. In both cases there are summations of internal forces reciprocally related to each other. The summations of internal forces generated on land are developed against and with the pull of gravity. The internal force in the water is accomplished by pulling or pushing against the resistance created by the water itself. This interaction between summation of internal forces developed on land and in the water is commonly observed during the racing start in a competitive swimming meet.

To obtain maximum propulsive force in the water, a broad surface must be presented by the moving limbs and by exerting a backward pressure in the water through a range of motion consistent with the desired execution of the stroke. (*Surface area for propulsive force*) The propulsive force which propels the body in the desired direction should be performed to avoid counteracting forces which would tend to retard linear motion in the water. For example, excessive hip flexion during the dolphin kick of the "butterfly stroke" would create undesired forces that would impede the desirable propulsive forces created by the upper limbs during the stroke (Figure 10.8). In this example, excessive hip flexion would present a broader surface area, but it would be in direct opposition to the desired linear motion of the butterfly stroke. Propulsive

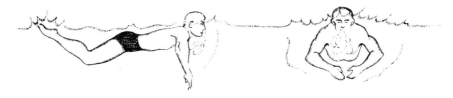

Figure 10.8. Surface area propulsive force. (After Counsilman, 1968.)

forces executed during any swimming stroke must be timed and sequential to bring about the desired summation of internal forces. This does not differ appreciably from the summation of internal forces generated during a skill on land.

External resistance in a water medium differs from external resistance on land. Gravity and air resistance are the primary external resistance forces on land. In contrast, the external resistance for the performer in the water comes from the water itself, the physical characteristics of the body to the water, and the movement of the water in an undesired fashion. (*Water resistance*)

One drag or resistance factor provided by the water is viscosity. (*Water viscosity*) All fluids have a greater or lesser degree of viscosity. In relation to other fluids, water has a small amount of viscosity; consequently, viscosity is relatively unimportant for the swimmer. However, it must be considered when swimming in salt water. Viscosity is the property in fluid which resists flow. Salt water, while providing more buoyancy for the swimmer, is more viscous than fresh water. Speed records in salt water would be slower than speed records in fresh water. This would be due primarily to the differences in viscosity.

The streamlined body tends to be more conducive to speed swimming because it presents less resistance to the water owing to its linear shape as opposed to a nonlinear, or bulky-type, body. Excessive body hair and bulky swimming apparel may very well have an adverse effect upon swimming speed since they add to the overall resistance of the body in the water.

As the body moves through water it creates water turbulence. This is a form of resistance with which the swimmer must cope as he moves through the water, especially in a closed pool. Water turbulence consists of waves, eddies, and low-pressure areas. These three factors also present drag or resistance on the swimmer. Waves and eddies are reduced by eliminating as many extraneous motions as possible. (*Waves*) They can be reduced further by keeping the body and its parts submerged as much as possible, consistent with the stroke being performed. Furthermore, eddies can be reduced somewhat by filling a pool above the drain gutters. (*Eddies*) Low-pressure areas are seen immediately behind the swimmer. (*Low-pressure area*) Excessive and extraneous motions of the limbs tend to generate a greater low-pressure area immediately behind the swimmer. This creates a suction effect which retards the linear motion of the swimmer.

Water is used in some sports as a propelling factor and also as a stabilizing force. As an example of water being used to stabilize body parts, the water polo player must propel himself as high as possible out of the water in preparing himself to make a throw toward the goal.

When the throw is initiated, the lower limbs are stabilized by the water to allow the serape effect to occur as a part of the summation of internal forces. In various coastal regions of the world, body surfing is a sport. In this sport the surfer must present his entire body in a streamlined fashion, with as much surface area as possible, to the moving water or waves. The waves will propel him linearly toward the beach.

SELECTED REFERENCES

1. ALEXANDER, ROBER S. "Immediate Effects of Stretch on Muscle Contractility." *American Journal of Physiology* 196:807-810, April, 1959.
2. ALLEY, L. E. "An Analysis of Water Resistance and Propulsion in Swimming the Crawl Stroke." *Research Quarterly* 23:253, October, 1952.
3. BASS, RUTH. "A Study of the Mechanics of Graceful Walking." *Research Quarterly* 8:173-180, May, 1937.
4. BOWNE, MARY E. "Relationship of Selected Measures of Acting Body Levers to Ball Throwing Velocities." *Research Quarterly* 31:392-402, October, 1960.
5. BRINING, T. R. "Measuring Air Resistance in Running." *Athletic Journal* 11:32-34, 1941.
6. CURETON, T. K. "Mechanics and Kinesiology of Swimming." *Research Quarterly* 1:87, December, 1930.
7. ———. "Mechanics of the High Jump." *Scholastic Coach* 4:9, 1935.
8. ———. "Mechanics of the Broad Jump." *Scholastic Coach* 4:8, 1935.
9. ———. "Mechanics of the Shot Put." *Scholastic Coach* 4:7-10, March, 1935.
10. ———. "Mechanics of the Track Racing Start." *Scholastic Coach* 4:14-16, January, 1935.
11. ———. "Mechanics of Track Running." *Scholastic Coach* 4:7-10, February, 1935.
12. DYSON, GEOFFREY H. G. *The Mechanics of Athletics.* London: University of London Press, 1964.
13. ECKERT, HELEN M. "Linear Relationships of Isometric Strength to Propulsive Force, Angular Velocity and Angular Acceleration in the Standing Broad Jump." *Research Quarterly* 35:298-306, October, 1964.
14. ———. "A Concert of Force-Energy in Human Movement." *Physical Therapy* 45:213-218, March, 1965.
15. FLETCHER, J. G., LEWIS, H. E., and WILKIE, D. R. "Human Power Output: The Mechanics of Pole Vaulting." *Ergonomics* 3:30-34 and 89, 1960.
16. GANSLEN, RICHARD V. "The Science of Athletics." *Amateur Athlete,* October, 1941.
17. ———. "Aerodynamic Factors Which Influence Discus Flight." *Discobolus* 5:9-12, December, 1958.
18. GANSLEN, RICHARD V., and HALL, KENNETH G. *The Aerodynamics of Javeline Flight.* Fayetteville: University of Arkansas Press, 1960.
19. GARDNER, GERALD. "Mechanical Principles of Athletics." Unpublished Paper. University of Southern California, 1963.
20. GOLDSTEIN, ALVIN G. "Linear Acceleration and Apparent Distance." *Perceptual and Motor Skills* 9:267-269, September, 1959.

21. GROVES, W. H. "Mechanical Analysis of Diving." *Research Quarterly* 22, May, 1950.
22. HENRY, F. M. "The Velocity Curve of Sprint Running." *Research Quarterly* 23, December, 1951.
23. ———. "Force-time Characteristics of the Sprint Start." *Research Quarterly* 23:301, October, 1952.
24. HEUSNER, WILLIAM W. "Theoretical Specifications for the Racing Dive: Optimum Angle of Take-off." *Research Quarterly* 30:25-37, March, 1959.
25. KARPOVICH, P. V., and PESTRECOR, K. "Mechanical Work and Efficiency in Swimming Crawl and Back Strokes." *Arbeitsphysiologie* 10:504-514, 1939.
26. LANE, ELIZABETH C., and MITCHEM, JOHN C. "Buoyancy as Predicted by Certain Anthropometric Measurements." *Research Quarterly* 35:21-24, March, 1964.
27. LIBERSON, W. T. "Biomechanics of Gait: A Method Study." *Archives of Physical Medicine and Rehabilitation* 46:37-48, January, 1965.
28. LISSNER, HERBERT R. "Introduction to Biomechanics." *Archives of Physical Medicine and Rehabilitation* 46:2-9, January, 1965.
29. LUPTON, HARTLEY. "An Analysis of the Effects of Speed on the Mechanical Efficiency of Human Muscular Movement." *Journal of Physiology* LVII:337-353, 1923.
30. MARSHALL, STAN. "Factors Affecting Place Kicking in Football." *Research Quarterly* 29:302-308, October, 1958.
31. MOHR, DOROTHY R., and BARRETT, MILDRED E. "Effect of Knowledge of Mechanical Principles in Learning to Perform Intermediate Swimming Skills." *Research Quarterly* 33:574-580, December, 1962.
32. NATSOULAS, T. "Principles of Momentum and Kinetic Energy in Perception of Causality." *American Journal of Psychology* 74:394-402, September, 1961.
33. NELSON, RICHARD C. "Follow-up Investigation of the Velocity of the Volleyball Spike." *Research Quarterly* 35:83-84, March, 1964.
34. NICKEL, DAVID L., and ALLEN, B. L. "The Negro and Learning to Swim." *The Physical Educator* 26:28-29, March, 1969.
35. SANTSCHI, W. R., and OTHERS. "Moment of Inertia and Centers of Gravity of the Living Human Body." *Technical Documentary Report* No. AMRL-TDR-63-36 Wright Patterson Air Force Base, Ohio, May, 1963.
36. SELIN, CARL. "An Analysis of the Aerodynamics of Pitched Baseball." *Research Quarterly* 30:228-232, May, 1959.
37. SHATEL, A. "Scientific Principles of Wrestling Skills." *Scholastic Coach* 32:72-75, 1961.
38. SLATER-HAMMELL, A. T. "Velocity Measurement of Fast Balls and Curve Balls." *Research Quarterly* 23:95, March, 1952.
39. SLOCUM, D. B., and BOWERMAN, W. "The Biomechanics of Running." *Clinical Orthopedics* 23:39-45, 1962.
40. SPENCER, RICHARD R. "Ballistics in the Mat Kip." *Research Quarterly* 34:213-218, May, 1963.
41. SUTTON, R. M. "Two Notes on the Physics of Walking." *American Journal of Physics* 32:490-491, 1955.
42. WHITING, H. T. A. "Variations in Floating Ability with Age in the Female." *Research Quarterly* 36:216-218, May, 1965.

43. WHITLEY, J. D., and SMITH, L. E. "Velocity Curves and Static Strength-Action Strength Correlations in Relation to the Mass Moved by the Arm." *Research Quarterly* 34:379-395, October, 1963.
44. WHITNEY, R. J. "Mechanics of Normal Muscular Activity." *Nature* 181: 942-944, 1958.
45. WINTER, F. W. "Mechanics of the Tuck Position in Executing the Forward Three and One-Half Somersault." *Athletic Journal* 45:19, January, 1965.

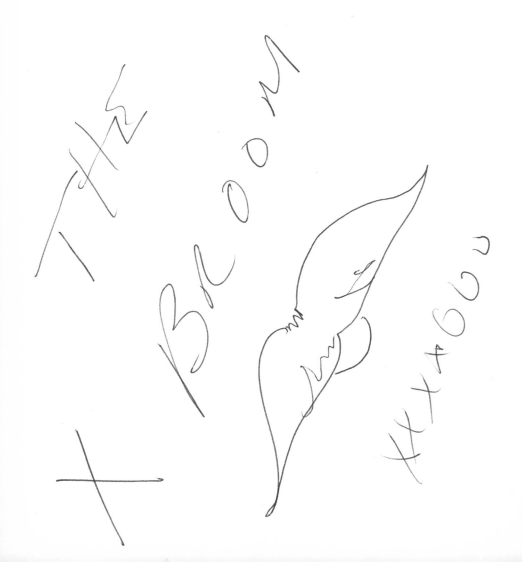

analytic kinesiology techniques

Teaching neuromuscular skills is based on (1) the analytic ability of the physical educator and (2) the ability to communicate pertinent facets of skill analyses to learners. *Analysis is the beginning point for teaching. Communication of the analytic information to the learner is teaching.* The techniques of skill analyses are learned, in part, by the future physical educator in one phase of undergraduate professional preparation called analytic kinesiology. The study of analytic kinesiology includes a merger of kinesiologic theory with practical aspects of sport techniques. The latter is usually learned in sport theory classes. The individual also learns about the technical aspects of sport and dance by performing. Performance is a vital aspect of professional preparation in physical education.

Better coaches throughout the world, especially in track and swimming, use cinematographic analyses as the basis for most of their on-the-field or in-the-pool coaching, i. e., coaching suggestions for skill development and coaching plans are derived after viewing films of athletes competing. This gives their work on the field and elsewhere greater significance, because these coaches have actually studied the athlete kinesiologically during a performance, and the coaching suggestions are designed specifically to correct the athlete's major problem. *The better coaches at all education and athletic levels incorporate scientific knowledge in their coaching.*

It is not uncommon to observe a "coach" watching an athlete attempt a skill once. The athlete is then given extensive information regarding the performance faults. There are at least two major factors to consider in such a case: (1) There is variability among performances by the same performer executing a skill. It is entirely possible that a coach may not see a consistent or major problem during one trial; (2) A discussion of all the athlete's faults related to a given skill will only tend to confuse and discourage him or impede motor learning. Like the physician who will not give medication to his patient because it may mask symptoms and prevent accurate diagnosis, the physical educator must observe a given athletic performance several times to see if major faults (symptoms) are occurring consistently. When the physical educator is sure he has the problem(s) "diagnosed," he can then "prescribe" activities designed specificially to improve the performance of the athlete. Guesswork and a lack of knowledge about the performer and the athletic performance could be "fatal," i. e., a coach who is lethargic, professionally apathetic, and unaware of kinesiologic techniques is not as likely to improve performances in his athletes as a coach who utilizes his scientific knowledge in teaching.

As stated above, physical educators must rely on their abilities to analyze athletic performances and make corrections in performance based on their analytic abilities without the use of motion picture film or video tape. This necessitates the development of a high level of sensitivity to determine what is *actually* occurring within the performance. The physical educator's sensitivity for looking at performances can be heightened by developing a systematic procedure for observing human motion. This is especially important when working without the assistance of cinematographic equipment.

▶ Noncinematographic Techniques

For best results, athletic performance should be analyzed within the competitive situation. If this is not possible, the athlete should perform for analysis purposes in gamelike situations. Too much conscious awareness of being analyzed might distort performance. If the performer realizes that analysis is occurring, he may perform differently from the way he performs during competition. This human trait must be considered during the analysis procedure.

To analyze a sport skill, the athlete should perform the skill several times before teaching or coaching suggestions are made. There are various ways in which a physical educator can observe human motion. The following systematic approach to observing sport skills is based on viewing body segments specifically during the performance. This *segmental approach* to observing sport skills is applicable to cinematographic analysis as well as noncinematographic analysis. Experience has indicated that a performer should be observed a minimum of eight times prior to making any teaching suggestions. The observations for each trial would be to observe the (1) total performance, (2) pelvic area and rib cage, (3) base of support or feet, (4) head and shoulders, (5) arm and hand,

(6) knees and hips, (7) follow-through, and (8) total performance once again. (Rose, 1959) The questions following are examples of the type that should be asked and ultimately answered. It should be noted that questions would differ depending upon the skill under observation; consequently, the physical educator should make a check list for each skill under study. Examples of this systematic, segmental analysis technique are found in Chapter 12.

OBSERVATIONS

I. Total Performance
   A. What is the general timing on the part of the athlete for the total skill?
   B. What was the outcome of the performance?

II. Pelvic Area and Rib Cage. The center of gravity is a relatively slow movement area and a good orientation point for analysis when compared to limb actions.
   A. How high is the center of gravity from its base?
   B. What is the critical path for center of gravity movement?
   C. Does the critical path change during any phase of the movement?
   D. What is the extent and direction of the total pelvic action?

III. Base of Support
   A. How does the body weight shift at the start, during, and finish of action?
   B. What is the line of projection for efficient action? *angle of arm*
   C. Does the *angle* line of projection during the performance change?
   D. In what direction(s) do the feet point prior to, during, and at the completion of the performance?
   E. Are the feet too wide or too close together during the performance?
   F. What is the position of the feet immediately prior to the action?

IV. Head and Shoulders
   A. Is the head in the proper position at the start, during, and at the end of the action?
   B. Are both eyes focused on the objective?
   C. What is the preferred eye of the performer?
   D. Were the eyes open or closed during the crucial phase of the performance?

    E. Is there any abnormal movement at the start of the performance which would have an adverse effect on subsequent movements?

    F. In cases where an implement is used, are the eyes focused on the object to be hit at the moment of impact?

  V. Arm and Hand

    A. In what direction do the arms move during the action?

    B. Are the arms too close or too far from the body for effective movement?

    C. Are the arms moving diagonally or in flexion-extension patterns?

    D. In cases where an implement is used, is the proper grip taken initially and held throughout the performance?

    E. In cases of impact, was the implement released at the point of impact?

    F. Was the total range of motion of both arms adequate?

    G. Are both arms rotated properly?

  VI. Knees and Hips

    A. In what direction do the legs move during the action?

    B. Are the knee flexion angles consistent with the skill to be performed?

    C. Are there any rotational movements at the hips which might inhibit performance?

    D. Is there any indication of inadequate flexibility at the hip joints?

    E. If impact is an integral part of the skill, what are the knee and hip actions immediately prior to, during, and following impact?

    F. Are the legs moving diagonally or in flexion-extension patterns?

  VII. Follow-through and/or Recovery

    A. What is the extent, direction, and pattern of the follow-through?

    B. Is there any evidence that muscular tension impeded the follow-through? If so, in what body segments?

    C. If an implement was used, how did it react at the point of impact and during the follow-through?

    D. Was the follow-through continuous?

    E. Was the recovery related to subsequent movements?

  VIII. Total Performance

    A. Was there an effective summation of internal forces?

    B. Was the objective of the skill met?

Following the study of these observations, several faults will undoubtedly be observed in the average performance. These will need to be corrected in order to improve the individual's overall performance. One important human trait must be considered: *Man usually concentrates on one thing at a time.* This means that the physical educator should not initially disclose all analytic findings to the athlete.

Teaching takes place following the analysis. The physical educator must use his professional judgment to place the athlete's performance faults on a priority list, i. e., the most flagrant fault must head the list, and other faults would be listed in diminishing order of performance. The most serious fault should receive immediate attention. The physical educator should give the athlete help in the form of *specific* changes in technique, body mechanics, skill drills, developmental exercises, or whatever is indicated to correct the most serious fault and ultimately improve the athlete's performance. This should be communicated to the athlete in language that he can understand, not necessarily in detailed scientific or kinesiologic terminology. When the athlete's major performance problem has been corrected, the second fault on the priority list should receive the same degree of attention.

Coaching suggestions must be specific for each athlete. Some coaches tend to frustrate their athletes. For example, a baseball coach who tells the hitter who has been in a "slump" that he needs to hit the ball more often is adding insult to injury. That type of generalization is absolutely useless, but unfortunately, some people and administrators call it teaching or coaching. The athlete in this example does not need to be told to hit the ball. He needs to be analyzed kinesiologically and his faults determined; and subsequently he must be helped to correct those faults. That is teaching-coaching.

▶ Cinematographic Techniques

Cinematography involves the use of the camera to record motion for subsequent kinesiologic analyses. Cameras used for cinematographic analyses range from still cameras through sophisticated motor-driven, high-speed motion picture cameras. The physical educator should view the film produced by these cameras in essentially the same way he would observe motion by means of noncinematographic techniques.

Analyzing a performance by means of film has a decided advantage over analysis with the unaided eye. For example, film can be studied frame-by-frame on a stop-action projector. This enables the physical educator to critically evaluate every aspect of the performance which may not have been observed with the unaided eye during the actual performance. In addition, cinematographic techniques allow the physical educator to make relatively accurate measurements of joint movements, as well as velocity of the body and its moving parts, directly from the projected image. Because of these advantages and others, the use of cinematographic techniques is essential in the teaching-coaching process.

Most institutions have available audiovisual materials such as cameras, projectors, microfilm readers, editor-viewers, and other pieces of photographic paraphernalia. Consequently, the tools are available for cinematographic analysis purposes. If photographic equipment is not available, there are relatively inexpensive cameras and projectors on the market, both of the eight millimeter and sixteen millimeter variety.

CAMERAS—Whether or not to use eight millimeter or sixteen millimeter equipment depends primarily upon funds and equipment available. Sixteen millimeter is preferred over eight millimeter equipment for cinematographic analysis for at least two reasons: (1) obviously, the image is larger and provides greater detail and (2) most educational institutions are equipped to work with sixteen millimeter as opposed to eight millimeter film. Some institutions do not provide cinematographic equipment for their personnel; consequently, the physical educator who employs cinematographic techniques will usually purchase eight millimeter cinematograhpic equipment for his personal use. Analyses can be made professionally, and money can be saved.

It is recommended that the camera have variable speeds up to sixty-four frames per second for analysis purposes. Cinematographic analysis can be done effectively by using thirty-two to sixty-four frames per second during the filming process. Film taken at less than thirty-two frames per second will be too blurred during maximum velocity performances of the limbs. There will be some blurring in film taken at thirty-two and sixty-four frames per second, but it is not enough to preclude its use. Film taken at thirty-two frames per second will permit the user to visualize the movement occurring frame-by-frame while observing the film with a stop-action projector. The gross perception of movement occurring within various body segments is less pronounced as the frames per second are increased. Also, it is economically more feasible to use thirty-two or sixty-four frames-per-second camera settings.

An interchangeable lens system is also recommended on a camera used for cinematographic analyses purposes. A telephoto lens with "zoom" capabilities is of particular importance. The use of a telephoto lens will reduce the amount of parallax. Parallax involves a perspective error when the camera is relatively close to the subject being filmed. The telephoto lens will reduce this error by enabling the photographer to be farther from the photographed subject. Perspective errors are recorded by the camera lens because it does not have the ability to make size adjustments like the human eye. The human makes automatic perspective adjustments with the eyes as he moves closer to or farther from the object. This is a learned phenomenon, and it has not been duplicated in camera lenses. An ideal camera with a multiple lens apparatus should have the following f stops: (1) The standard lens should have a f stop range from 1.9 to 22; (2) The wide-angle lens should have f stop settings from 1.8 to 16; and (3) The telephoto lens should have an f stop setting from 2.5 to 32. This combination of lenses will provide efficient film-making for types of film speeds recommended and varying light conditions.

Several factors must be considered prior to photographing the subject to be analyzed. These include the position of the camera relative to the performer, the height of the camera in relation to the center of mass of the individual to be filmed, the actual distance of the camera from the performance, the size of the performer in relation to the view finder, and the time taken to perform the skill. *If only one sequence is to be filmed, the camera should be placed at a ninety-degree angle to the most important movement plane of motion.*

For analytic purposes, multiple views are preferred. Ideally, these should be taken from the side, front, back, and above the performer. Photographing two views of the same subject on one frame can be accomplished by using a dichroic mirror and photographing the individual from above, from the side, or from the front. (Cooper and Sorani, 1965) To further reduce distortions, the height of the camera should be centered on the object to be photographed. To maintain a constant level as well as stability for the camera, it is recommended that a stable tripod be used during the photographic process. It is difficult to control the distance of the camera from the performing subject, especially when the subject is filmed during an athletic contest. However, it is essential to have at least one known distance for future reference when analyzing the film. It is also important to have an actual measurement of some part of the performer. For example, the length of the forearm might be measured between two anatomic landmarks. This can be used for future reference to assist the observer in determining the velocity of linear motion as well as the actual size of the object in various positions and the range of motion of the joints involved. When the size of a body part is known, the projected image can be scaled to determine its actual size.

Timing within films is another very essential aspect. There is disparity between cameras because some cameras are motor-driven while other cameras are spring-driven. The timing factor is relatively constant in motor-driven cameras as opposed to spring-driven cameras. Motor-driven cameras are expensive; consequently, they are not used as frequently for cinematographic purposes as the less expensive spring-driven cameras. To insure accuracy in timing when using spring-driven cameras, it is essential to include a timing device in the analysis film. The timing device should be a clock readable to .01 of a second. This will serve as a check on the accuracy of the frames-per-second setting of the camera. If it is not possible to include a timing device in a film, the operator of the spring-driven camera should take care to have maximum tension on the spring mechanism by having it fully wound before each photographic session.

Ultra-high-speed cameras are available for cinematographic research purposes. These motor-driven cameras have special sprocket systems which allow filming of athletic performances within the range of 100 to 32,000 frames per second. Obviously, the use of this type of camera is unrealistic for the average person interested in using film analysis in school situations.

Cameras are also available with stroboscopic light attachments. This type of camera gives the individual a sequential multiple image on one photographic print. Some of these cameras will produce multiple pictures of the same performance on separate photographs. The multiple image and instant developing features on this camera are useful tools in the analysis-teaching process. However, it has the disadvantage of producing a relatively small image.

There are photographic equipment accessories which should be included to insure adequate results during the filming process. It is recommended that the camera be purchased with a good light meter system built into it. This will avoid many filming difficulties, especially for the novice photographer. To insure good pictures indoors, it is advisable to have at least five photo floods on stands strategically placed during photographic sessions. It is recommended that the floods be placed as follows: (1) two on both sides at forty-five-degree angles, knee level to the performer; (2) two on both sides at forty-five-degree angles, chest level to the performer, and (3) one high enough to spotlight the head. These would be of particular value to coaches in such sports as basketball, wrestling, and gymnastics. However, photo floods are of little practical value during the filming of an actual contest since they would be in the way.

It is essential to provide a known measurement in the background of films used for cinematographic analysis. One way of doing this is to photograph a subject in an athletic practice situation and include a portable gird screen in the background. A grid screen can be constructed from 4 feet by 8 feet Masonite or plyboard panels. Tempered Masonite is recommended because it is lighter in physical weight than plyboard. The grid squares should be at least four inches marked off in contrasting colors with lines no less than one-eighth inch in width. The overall size of the total grid screen would depend upon the athletic skill to be photographed. It must be remembered that there will be a slight amount of perspective error when using a grid screen; consequently, it should be used only as a rough guide for a known measurement.

The problem of having a known background measure is more difficult when filming during an actual athletic contest. However, there is usually one part of the physical surroundings which can be measured prior to or following the filming in order to provide a known measurement. This might be a part of the stands, a goalpost, or other constant aspects within the surroundings.

PROJECTORS—Several essential criteria must be considered prior to selecting a motion analysis projector: (1) single frame stop-action with the ability to hold a picture indefinitely without film damage from heat; (2) single frame-by-frame advance feature without flicker; (3) forward and reverse capabilities at multiple speeds; (4) constant illumination; (5) constant focus; (6) a frame counter that will add, subtract, and reset; and (7) a remote control allowing the operator to control all speeds, stop-action, and forward and reverse motion. Although motion analysis can be done with regular and slow-motion projectors, the features listed above are needed to perform a complete analysis. Eight millimeter and sixteen millimeter projectors which include these features are available at a relatively low cost.

Another piece of photographic equipment which can be used to analyze film at a low-budget level is the editor-viewer. There are several models available to accommodate eight millimeter and sixteen millimeter film. The major consideration in regard to film analysis is the size of the projected image on the viewing screen. The screens on editor-viewers are built into the total apparatus; consequently, the size of the projected image cannot be changed. A good editor-viewer is a recommended piece of equipment, even though a high-quality motion analysis projector is available. The editor-viewer will permit editing, splicing, and preparing film for the library.

Microfilm readers may also be used for motion analysis purposes. One limitation of the microfilm reader is that the projected image cannot be enlarged or reduced as needed.

For sophisticated motion analysis research, there are very expensive motion analyzers available. Essentially, these motion analysis units consist of a projector and angle measurement read-out screen which works automatically to gather data and feed these data into a computerized system for analysis purposes. This computerized unit can be programmed to provide an automatic read-out of all visible joint movements performed by the subject being analyzed.

FILM—The choice of film for analysis is dependent upon the nature of the desired outcome. Film makers are constantly improving their products. The choice of film, therefore, should be based upon the camera used, film speeds, lighting conditions, and the ultimate objective for use of the film. For analysis purposes, black-and-white film is preferred to colored film since better contrasts are seen in black-and-white film. However, if the film is to be used within a class for instructional purposes in order to illustrate a kinesiologic principle, color film might well be used.

FILM ANALYSIS—Once the film has been processed, it should be observed several times at regular speed. Following these general observations, the film should be analyzed frame-by-frame, using the noncinematographic segmental techniques discussed earlier in this chapter. This requires a minimum of eight separate frame-by-frame observations of the performer's body segments. During these analysis observations, notes should be made on specific segmental and joint movements.

For specific joint analysis, there are two general techniques that may be employed. These may be done in conjunction with each other or separately. The most commonly used technique is a tracing of the *contour* or body outline on paper (Figures 12.4–12.12). A workable image size should be projected and drawn. For individual contour drawings, 8 1/2-by-11-inch paper is adequate. These drawings can be done on transparencies approximately the same size for subsequent projection using an overhead projector. The advantage of the transparency is that the total number of drawings may be superimposed for multiple-image projection. Artistic ability is not essential for this process; however, the tracing should be accurate enough to determine joint angles. It should be reemphasized, however, that attainment of absolute joint angles is impossible with photographic techniques, due primarily to perspective error. However, enough joint angle accuracy can be determined to conduct a cinematographic analysis. The second analysis procedure is called the *point-and-line* technique. In this technique, a point is used to indicate the center of a joint or anatomic landmark, and the lines that connect these points indicate body segments. It is essential that one of the points be utilized to indicate the center of the pelvic segment. This can be used to make an estimate of the line of movement, or parabola. This technique provides a less cluttered multi-image picture and more accurate joint angle measurements (Figures 12.13 and 12.14). On the other hand, the image of the performer is lost.

It is obvious that doing a contour drawing or a point-and-line drawing of every frame is unnecessary. There are two suggested ways for selecting frames to be analyzed and drawn. First, a decision should be made based on the number of total frames analyzed for the skill under study. For example, if the total skill consists of thirty-two frames and eight drawings are desired, this would mean that every fourth frame will be drawn. This procedure has the advantage of a consistent time interval between drawings. The second procedure consists of determining *crucial phases* of the performance after the film has been observed several times. This technique actually places the emphasis at the crucial points of the skill where the performer's faults may be more obvious. Using the first procedure, a crucial movement might be missed. To assist in the subsequent analysis, the frame number should be included on each drawing.

TELEVISION EQUIPMENT—Use of television and video tape for cinematographic analysis purposes has potential. There are three pieces of television equipment necessary for kinesiologic analysis. These are a video camera, video recorder, and video monitor-receiver. The overall cost of these three items is comparable to an adequate camera and projector for motion analysis.

There are several advantages of video tape over eight millimeter or sixteen millimeter film. The major advantage lies in the fact that video tape can be taken of a performer and replayed instantly for analysis purposes. In addition, and adding to the instant replay, is the fact that verbal comments can be recorded simultaneously with the video tape. To do the same thing with film is impractical. Instant video tape and sound recording are very useful from analysis and teaching standpoints. For example, the athlete can be shown his major problems immediately. The coach can make specific teaching suggestions to help the athlete improve his skill level. The coach can record his noncinematographic observations verbally while he is videotaping the athlete's performance initially. These spontaneous remarks by the coach can be retained and used later in a more detailed approach to the analysis. This means that the coach can make a more functional use of the observation check list.

There are other advantages to the use of video tape. The light is a less crucial factor, video tape is less expensive than most film, and all television cameras are motor-driven. There are no spring-driven television cameras with the inconsistent speed factor. The television camera does not have a frame-by-frame timing element as does a sixteen millimeter or eight millimeter camera; however, video tape does move through the camera at a set rate of inches per second. The inches-per-second recording is made on the video tape recorder, and this information can be utilized to assist in the timing process of the kinesiologic analysis. For further timing accuracy a .01 of a second clock can be included in the televised picture. Since video tape does have some advantages over eight millimeter or sixteen millimeter film, it should be used for kinesiologic analyses and instructional purposes.

The television camera should be portable and capable of filming athletic performances in a wide variety of situations. It should have a preset speed device to allow video tape to move at a preset speed in inches per second through the camera. The camera should be fully automatic in regard to its video- and audio-level controls.

The most important item of television equipment for analytic purposes is the video tape recorder. It is absolutely essential that this piece of equipment have full-stop motion features. It should slow motion and have instant playback capabilities both in forward and reverse. Furthermore, video tape and audio channels should be capable of operation by remote control.

The television monitor-receiver should be a lightweight, portable unit. It should have quality video input and output systems as well as audio input and output systems. It is recommended that the minimum diagonal screen size for analysis purposes be eighteen inches.

The standard television equipment operates at one-thirtieth frames per second, that is, each frame is on the screen one-thirtieth of a second. In ballistic movements, this results in a blurred image. Special video tape recorders are available which have been developed for instant replay usage. These are capable of stopping very fast action. The major disadvantage of the equipment is that it limits the recording to twenty seconds. The recording is made on a metal drum rather than video tape. If regular television equipment is to be used, a stroboscopic light may be used to aid in stopping the action. However, this does require a darkened area or televising at night.

Selected References

1. Battye, C. K., and Joseph, J. "An Investigation of Telemetering of the Activity of Some Muscles in Walking." *Medical and Biological Engineering* 4:125-135, March, 1966.
2. Bierman, W., and Yamshon, L. J. "Electromyography in Kinesiologic Evaluations." *Archives of Physical Medicine* 29:206-211, 1948.
3. Cooper, John M., and Sorani, Robert P. "Use of the Dichroic Mirror as a Cinematographic Aid in the Study of Human Performance." *Research Quarterly* 36:210-211, May, 1965.
4. Cureton, T. K. "Elementary Principles and Techniques of Cinematographic Analysis." *Research Quarterly* 10:3, May, 1939.
5. Davis, Rober, Wehrkamp, Robert, and Smith, Karl U. "Dimensional Analysis of Motion: I. Effects of Laterality and Movement Direction." *Journal of Applied Psychology* 35:363-366, October, 1951.
6. Deshon, Deans E., and Nelson, Richard C. "A Cinematographical Analysis of Sprint Running." *Research Quarterly* 35:451-455, December, 1964.
7. De Vries, Herbert A. "A Cinematographical Analysis of the Dolphin Swimming Stroke." *Research Quarterly* 30, No. 4:413-422, December, 1959.
8. Dunwoody, Katherine M. "Time and Motion in Physical Education." *Journal of Health and Physical Education* 10:218-220; 263, April, 1939.

9. FALLS, HAROLD B., JR. ed. *Exercise Physiology.* New York: Academic Press, Inc., 1968.
10. FENN, W. O. "Mechanical Energy Expenditure in Sprint Running as Measured by Moving Pictures." *American Journal of Physiology* 90:343-344, 1929.
11. FLINT, M. MARILYN. "Lumbar Posture: A Study of Roentgenographic Measurement and the Influence of Flexibility and Strength." *Research Quarterly* 34:15-20, March, 1963.
12. GOLLNICK, PHILIP D., and KARPOVICH, PETER V. "Electrogoniometric Study of Locomotion and Some Athletic Movements." *Research Quarterly* 35:357-369, October, 1964.
13. HARTSON, L. D. "Analysis of Skilled Movements." *Personnel Journal* 11:28-43, 1932-1933.
14. ———. "Contrasting Approaches to the Analysis of Skilled Movements." *Journal of General Psychology* 20:263-293, April, 1939.
15. HELLEBRANDT, F. A., HELLEBRANDT, E. J., and WHITE, CLARENCE H. "Methods of Recording Movement." *American Journal of Physical Medicine* 39:178-183, October, 1960.
16. HERMANN, GEORGE W. "Electromyographic Study of Selected Muscles Involved in the Shot Put." *Research Quarterly* 33:85-93, March, 1962.
17. HUBBARD, A. W. "Experimental Analysis of Running and of Certain Fundamental Differences Between Trained and Untrained Runners." *Research Quarterly* 10:28, 1939.
18. HUBBARD, ALFRED W., and SENG, CHARLES N. "Visual Movements of Batters." *Research Quarterly* 25:42-57, March, 1954.
19. HUBBARD, ALFRED W., and STETSON, R. H. "An Experimental Analysis of Human Locomotion." *American Journal of Physiology* 124:300-313, 1938.
20. KARPOVICH, PETER V., and GOLLNICK, PHILIP D. "Electrogonometric Study of Locomotion and Some Athletic Movements." *Federation Proceedings Abstracts* 21:313, March-April, 1962.
21. KELLIHER, M. S. "Analysis of Two Styles of Putting." *Research Quarterly* 34:344-349, October, 1963.
22. KING, W. H., and IRWIN, L. W. "A Time and Motion Study of Competitive Backstroke Swimming Turns." *Research Quarterly* 28:257-268, October, 1957.
23. KING, WILLIAM H., and SCHARF, RAPHAEL J. "Time and Motion Analysis of Competitive Freestyle Swimming Turns." *Research Quarterly* 35:37-44, March, 1964.
24. KITZMAN, ERIC W. "Baseball: Electromyographic Study of Batting Swing." *Research Quarterly* 35:166-178, May, 1964.
25. KLISSOURAS, VASSILIS, and KARPOVICH, PETER V. "Electrogoniometric Study of Jumping Events." *Research Quarterly* 38:41-48, March, 1967.
26. LAPP, V. W. "An Analysis of Movement on the Basis of Latent Times and Variabilities." *Research Quarterly* 6:19, October, 1935.
27. LOCKHART, AILEENE. "The Value of the Motion Picture as an Instructional Device in Learning a Motor Skill." *Research Quarterly* 15:181-187, May, 1944.
28. MASTROPAOLO, JOSEPH A. "Analysis of Fundamentals of Fencing." *Research Quarterly* 30:285-291, October, 1959.

29. MOSTERD, W. L., and JONGBLUED, J. "Analysis of the Stroke of Highly Trained Swimmers." *Arbeitsphysiologie* 20:288-293, 1964.
30. O'CONNELL, A. L., and GARDNER, E. B. "The Use of Electromyography in Kinesiological Research." *Research Quarterly* 34:166-184, May, 1963.
31. PAULY, JOHN E., and STEELE, RUSSELL W. "Electromyographic Analysis of Back Exercises for Paraplegic Patients." *Archives of Physical Medicine and Rehabilitation* 47:730-736, November, 1966.
32. PLAGENHOEF, S. C. "Methods for Obtaining Kinetic Data to Analyze Human Motions." *Research Quarterly* 34:103, March, 1966.
33. ROCK, I., TAUBER, E. S., and HELLER, D. P. "Perception of Stroboscopic Movement." *Science* 147:1050-1051, February, 1965.
34. ROSE, JACK. "Analysis of Track and Field Performances." Unpublished paper. California State College at Long Beach, 1959.
35. RUBIN, GERALD, VON TREBA, PATRICIA, and SMITH, KARL U. "Dimensional Analysis of Motion: II. Complexity of Movement Pattern." *Journal of Applied Psychology* 36:272-276, 1952.
36. SMITH, K. U., and GREENE, D. "Scientific Motion Study and Aging Processes in Performance." *Ergonomics* 5:155-164, January, 1962.
37. WEHRKAMP, ROBERT A., and SMITH, KARL U. "Dimensional Analysis of Motions: II. Travel-Distance Effects." *Journal of Applied Psychology* 36:201-206, June, 1936.

skill analysis phases

It has been emphasized throughout this book that kinesiology is one of the major "working tools" of the physical educator. The "key" to the quality of theoretical subject matter is whether or not it can be functionally applied in practice. If theory cannot be applied in practice, it is not good theory. Kinesiologic theory has withstood the test of time. By using it as a "working tool" in practice, the physical educator can help the individual student attain his potential as a performer. *This chapter is designed to serve as a model to show how kinesiologic theory can contribute to the teaching-coaching process.*

The six sequential phases listed below are recommended as a procedure for making analyses of athletic performances:

1. Gross observations of the performer.
2. Noncinematographic segmental analysis.
3. Cinematographic segmental analysis.
4. Aggregate muscular analysis.
5. Synthesis of kinesiologic constructs and myologic elements.
6. Prescribed recommendations for skill improvement.

▶ 1. Gross Observations of the Performer

The initial contact with the athletic squad or physical education class involves a subjective visual impression of the skill level of the performers within the squad or class. At this time, the physical educator makes some intuitive general "hunches" about the skill level of the individuals being observed. The students can be categorized as being good, average, or poor performers. But subjective impressions should be objectified. The degree to which this can be done is based upon the physical educator's professional preparation in the scientific foundations of physical education, his athletic experiences, and the quality of his professional preparation in the technical aspects of sport.

Since this first analysis phase is rather superficial, it should be understood that further steps in the analytic process are needed to provide professional bases for the improvement of performance. Unfortunately, many coaches without professional preparation in physical education do not go beyond this phase in attempting to improve sport performance. Nor does this initial observation give the physical educator enough information about the performer to make a professional judgment regarding his abilities. The old adage that the "first impression is a lasting impression" can be detrimental in this context. The physical educator usually makes his subjective judgments on the basis of his own stereotype of what constitutes "good form" for the skill being observed. While this is basically good practice, it does have the potential of eliminating the athlete who might be an effective performer even though he executes the skill in an unorthodox manner. As examples, radical changes have been observed in the execution of the shot put and the high jump in past years. If the performers who initiated these changes in style had been observed by some coaches on the first days of practice, they might have been "cut" from the squad or had their styles changed to conform to the coaches' stereotype of "good form." Therefore, on this basis, the first impression can be somewhat misleading. Furthermore, when dealing with growing and developing athletes, it is important to consider the *potential* of the individual. During the growth process, there will be changes in the anatomic and neurologic interrelationships which result in an appearance of awkwardness in the teen-age student. Thus, the first analysis phase should not be used to exclude the individual performer. It should be applied rather for homogenous grouping purposes for further analysis and development of the performers.

▶ 2. Noncinematographic Segmental Analysis

A discussion of the noncinematographic segmental analysis technique is found in Chapter 11. This is a systematic approach to observing sport skills. It deals with viewing and focusing attention on body segments and joints during the sport performance. As suggested, a minimum of eight observations for each performance is recommended. Observe (1) total performance, (2) pelvic area and rib cage, (3) base of support or feet, (4) head and shoulders, (5) arms and hands, (6) knees and hips, (7) follow-through and/or recovery, and (8) total performance once again.

During these noncinematographic segmental observations, joint movements and other observations should be recorded as suggested in

Figure 12.1. Major joint movements are discussed in Chapter 2. Estimations should be made of joint movements most crucial to the phase being observed. The three major performance phases are (1) preparatory, (2) movement, and (3) follow-through and/or recovery. These were discussed in a model format in Chapter 10. In addition, the crucial

Name: _____ Height: _____ Weight: _____ Age: _____

Position: _____ Skill Analyzed: _____ Date: _____

Overall Rating: _____

Instructions: Numbers should be placed by the major faulty or extraneous *joint movements* observed. The most serious movement fault would receive a one, etc. Indications of other skill problems should also be noted which are related to the kinesiologic considerations on page 2 [Figure 12.2]. **SPECIFIC** coaching recommendations to improve the athlete's performance are to be made on page 3 [Figure 12.3] following the noncinematographic or cinematographic analysis. A carbon copy of page 3 is given to the athlete and the original copy is retained by the coach.

Body Segments and Joints	Preparatory Sequence Observations	Movement Sequence Observations	Follow-Through and Recovery Sequence Observations
Pelvic Girdle & Rib Cage			
Base of Support			
Head & Shoulders			
Arms & Hands			
Knee & Hip Joints			

Figure 12.1. Segmental analysis work sheet.

joint ranges of motion and planes of motion should be recorded. Estimation of joint movements should be made in terms of degrees. Planes of motion should be listed by name.

As indicated in the instructions for Figure 12.1, following the non-cinematographic analysis observations, numbers should be placed by the major faults of the performer. The most serious fault should receive primary consideration by the athlete and physical educator. Figure 12.2,

---

MUSCLES MOST INVOLVED:

   What muscle groups are most critical to properly execute the skill? What muscle groups are being used improperly?

SUMMATION OF INTERNAL FORCES:

Prepartory Phase

   Muscle length-force ratio
   Base of support stability
   Body equilibrium

Movement Phase

   Kinetic Chain
   Serape effect
   Dynamic Stabilization
   Progressive, sequential segment
      velocity
   Large to small muscle force transfer
   Force applied in correct direction
   Projection speed
   Combined linear-angular motions
   Conservation of angular momentum
   Limb or body deceleration
   Foot Contact at Projection
   Grip

Recovery Phase

   Follow-through intensity
   Directional change
   Force dissipation

AERODYNAMICS:

Angle of Projection

Flight Pattern

   Parabola
   Flight Velocity
   Air density
   Projectile's shape
   Flight angle
   Projectile's surface area
   Texture-friction factor
   Spin
   Flight Stability

Landing Pattern

   Angle of incidence
   Rebound
   Surface friction and
      resiliency
   Elasticity
   Striking Surface's
      shape
   Rebound surface area

HYDRODYNAMICS:

   Buoyancy
   Surface area for
      propulsive force

Water Resistance:

   Viscosity
   Waves
   Eddies
   Low pressure areas

Figure 12.2.   Kinesiologic consideration for analysis.

kinesiologic considerations, is designed primarily as a "recall check list" of the more important kinesiologic subject matter to be considered during the observations of athletic performance. The appropriate kinesiologic considerations within Figure 12.2 must be selected for the performance being analyzed, and prescribed coaching recommendations for performance improvement may be recorded on the form shown in Figure 12.3.

OFFSEASON AND PRESEASON CONDITIONING PROGRAM

NAME: _____ POSITION: _____

1. Specifics:

2. Skill Development Drills:

3. Strength Development Exercises:

4. Flexibility Development Exercises:

5. Muscular Endurance Exercises:

6. Cardiovascular Endurance Activities:

Figure 12.3. Prescribed coaching recommendations to improve performance.

The individual without cinematographic equipment would eliminate analysis phases three and four and proceed to phases five and six. Phase five is an important step in the analysis process. This is the time when the experienced practicing physical educator reflects on his observations during phases one and two. These reflections also serve as a basis for phase six. Experience has shown that many physical educators tend to omit phase five and make crucial decisions during their actual observations. This is a mistake because there has not been enough time for critical reflexion upon the observed performance. *To improve performance, some time must be set aside by the physical educator to critically think through the totality of the individual's performance.* This is the essence of phase five. Phase six, specific recommendations for skill improvement, is the practical application of phase five. Examples of phases five and six of two levels of performers are discussed in detail.

▶ **3. Cinematographic Segmental Analysis**

A discussion of cinematographic techniques is presented in Chapter 11. The analytic process described in phase two above should be used in the same manner during a cinematographic analysis.

Cinematographic analyses of two softball hitters with different levels of ability are presented herein to serve as a model. The male performer was an All-World selection, and the female performed on an intercollegiate softball team. This model involving the two softball hitters is continued through phases four, five, and six. *These analysis phases illustrate how kinesiologic theory can be practiced.*

In this model analysis, the world class performer is serving as the stereotype of softball-hitting form. The major objectives of this cinematographic analysis are to find the major faults of the intercollegiate performer and improve her softball hitting ability. (Schuble, 1969)

STANCE—In sport skills where appropriate, the starting stance must be considered in the analytic process. The initial softball hitting stances are shown in Figures 12.7 and 12.8. These are static, or nonmoving, body positions. The initial stance should not be confused with the preparatory phase. During the preparatory phase the performer is moving, and he is placing muscles most involved on stretch preparatory to bringing about more potential force in order to achieve better efficiency during the summation of internal forces. When comparing the stances of the two performers, it can be seen that the female performer has an excessive amount of radial flexion in both wrists. This causes the bat to be carried too high and behind her head. She also has an excessive amount of right shoulder abduction. This contributes to the bat being held too high. Both elbows are flexed more than needed for proper execution of the softball swing. These basic faults combined lead to another major fault which is discussed below. Furthermore, there is one other notable difference between the stances of the two performers—namely, in the weight distribution over the lower limbs. The male performer distributes his weight evenly over both lower limbs. On the other hand, the female performer has distributed her weight primarily on her right leg.

Figures 12.4 through 12.12 are contour drawings taken from sixteen millimeter film of the two performers. The images were projected on paper and traced. For the male, four key phases were selected. Excluding the stance, these phases are consistent with those outlined in Figure 12.1. For the female performer, it was necessary to draw an extra frame during the movement phase to illustrate a major fault in softball-hitting form. The selection of vital frames for contour drawings used during the analysis is arbitrary. The major criterion to use is the importance of the movement shown on a particular frame to the overall execution of the skill. If a visual representation is needed to show the comparative speed of movement between body parts, the point-and-line technique for illustrating motion is recommended. This is illustrated for both performers in Figures 12.13 and 12.14. The point-and-line technique should have a consistent time interval between each point-and-line drawing. This can be determined when camera speed is constant and known.

Motion between contour drawings is the important factor for study. Each contour drawing is selected from a film frame to show an efficient flow of motion during the execution of the skill under study. In essence, the arbitrarily selected phases or illustrations by contour drawings serve as key reference points for the total motion. The physical educator must be primarily concerned with the motion throughout the total skill performance instead of focusing attention on the static illustrative phases only. Segmental analysis is essential to understand complex body motions seen in a skill such as softball-hitting. Ultimately, however, the physical educator must deal with total motion, and this is done for this kinesiologic model during phase five of the analysis.

Joint motions are described from the preparation sequence to the movement sequence, and these movements are indicated under the *preparatory heading.* Joint motions from the movement sequence to the follow-through sequence are described under the *movement heading.* Joint motions during the follow-through or recovery sequence are described under the *follow-through heading.*

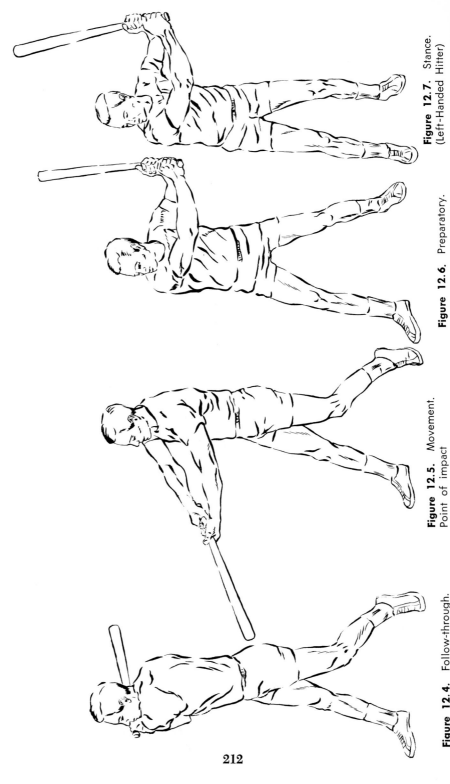

Figure 12.7. Stance. (Left-Handed Hitter)

Figure 12.6. Preparatory.

Figure 12.5. Movement. Point of impact

Figure 12.4. Follow-through.

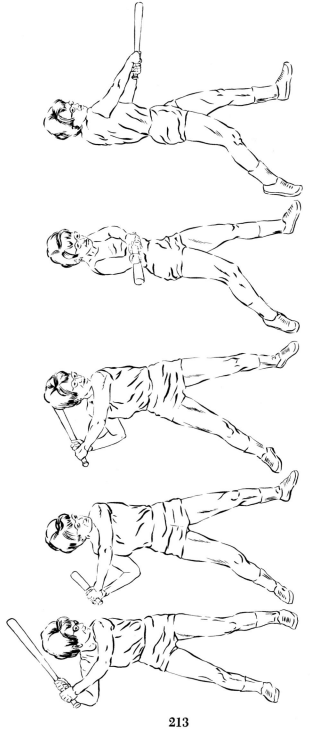

Figure 12.8. Stance. Right-handed hitter.

Figure 12.9. Preparatory. Start of "Hitch."

Figure 12.10. Preparatory—end of "Hitch."

Figure 12.11. Movement. Point of impact.

Figure 12.12. Follow-through.

213

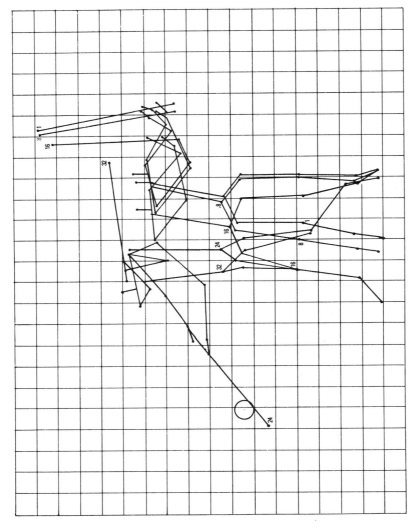

Figure 12.13. Point and line illustration—male performer. (Numbers indicate film frames. Film was taken at 32 frames/second.) Left handed hitter.

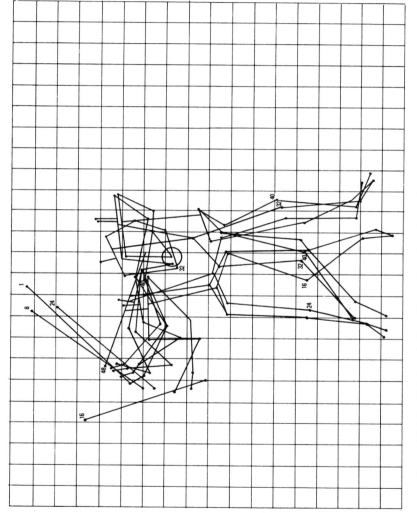

Figure 12.14. Point and line illustration—female performer. (Numbers indicate film frames. Film was taken at 32 frames/second.) Right handed hitter.

Preparatory Sequence

Figure 12.6

A. Pelvic girdle movements
   1. Slight right transverse rotation of the pelvic girdle.
B. Rib cage
   1. Slight spinal rotation, to the left of the lumbar and thoracic spines.
C. Base of support
   1. Right foot has moved approximately twelve inches in the direction of the pitcher.
   2. The toes of the right foot are pointed in the direction of the pitch as a result of right hip lateral rotation.
   3. The left foot remains relatively fixed.
D. Head and shoulders
   1. Slight cervical rotation to the right.
   2. Slight horizontal adduction of the right shoulder joint.

E. Arms and hands
   1. No change in the hands and wrist joints.

   2. The right elbow joint has extended slightly.
F. Knee and hip joints
   1. Slight lateral rotation of the right hip joint.
   2. Slight flexion of the right knee.
   3. Slight abduction at both hips.

Figure 12.9

A. Pelvic girdle movements
   1. Some left transverse pelvic rotation.
B. Rib cage
   1. Slight lumbar and thoracic rotation right.
C. Base of support
   1. Base of support has widened approximately twelve to fourteen inches.
   2. The left foot is moving to the left of the ball's line of flight. Slight lateral rotation and abduction of the left hip.
   3. Right foot remains relatively stable.
D. Head and shoulders
   1. Slight cervical rotation to the left.
   2. Slight left shoulder joint horizontal adduction and flexion.
   3. The right shoulder has adducted approximately twenty to twenty-five degrees. These movements have resulted in a drop of the bat from its original position in the stance.
E. Arms and hands
   1. The hands and wrists have maintained about the same position, but the bat is dropped due to shoulder action.
   2. There has been a slight extension of the left elbow.
F. Knee and hip joints
   1. Marked lateral rotation and flexion of the right knee.
   2. No change appreciable at right hip joint.
   3. Abduction and lateral rotation of the left hip joint.

Movement Sequence

Figure 12.10

A. (The female performer demonstrated a major fault at this point. Consequently, an extra frame was drawn to illustrate that fault, commonly known as a "hitch." The total "hitch" is illustrated between Figures 12.8 and 12.10.)

A. Pelvic girdle movements
1. Right transverse rotation continues.
B. Rib cage
1. Marked right lumbar and thoracic spinal rotation.
C. Base of support: no change.
D. Head and shoulders
1. Slight left cervical rotation.
2. Slight lateral flexion of the cervical spine.
3. Increased left shoulder flexion.
E. Arms and hands
1. Slight left elbow flexion.
2. Slight right shoulder abduction.
3. Slight right elbow flexion.
4. Hands remain the same.
F. Knee and hip joints
1. Medial rotation, right knee.
2. Abduction of the right hip.
3. Slight lateral rotation of the right hip.

Figure 12.5

A. Pelvic girdle movements
1. Approximately ninety degrees of right transverse pelvic girdle rotation.
B. Rib cage
1. Right thoracic spine rotation.

2. Slight left lateral flexion of the lumbar spine.
C. Base of support
1. Weight shift from the left foot to the right foot.
2. Plantar flexion of the left ankle joint.

Figure 12.11

A. Pelvic girdle movements
1. Ninety degrees of left transverse pelvic girdle rotation.
B. Rib cage
1. Considerable thoracic and lumbar spine rotation to the left.

C. Base of support
1. Weight shift to the left foot.

2. Plantar flexion of the right ankle.
3. No change in the width of the stance.

MALE PERFORMER	FEMALE PERFORMER

D. Head and shoulders
  1. Slight left cervical rotation.
  2. Left shoulder joint low, diagonal adduction and medial rotation.
  3. Right shoulder joint low, diagonal abduction and lateral rotation.
  4. The total motion of the arms and bat is through a low diagonal plane of motion.
	D. Head and shoulders
	  1. Right cervical rotation.
	  2. Slight cervical flexion.
	
	  3. Marked right shoulder joint diagonal adduction and medial rotation.
	  4. Marked left shoulder joint diagonal abduction and lateral rotation. The arms and bat are moving through low diagonal plane of motion.

E. Arms and hands
  1. Left elbow has moved from flexion to extension.
  2. The right elbow remains about the same.
  3. Both wrists are ulnar flexing.
	E. Arms and hands
	  1. Excessive left elbow flexion.
	  2. Extensive right elbow flexion.
	  3. Ulnar flexion starting at both wrists.

F. Knee and hip joints
  1. Slight right knee extension.
  2. Marked left knee flexion.
  3. Marked medial rotation of the right hip.
	F. Knee and hip joints
	  1. Moving into left knee extension.
	  2. Right knee flexion.
	  3. Medial rotation of the left hip.

Follow-Through or Recovery Sequence

MALE PERFORMER	FEMALE PERFORMER
Figure 12.4	**Figure 12.12**

A. Pelvic girdle movements
  1. Continuation of right transverse pelvic girdle rotation.
B. Rib cage
  1. Slight right lateral flexion of the lumbar spine.
  2. Continued thoracic spine rotation to the right.
C. Base of support
  1. Foot placement relatively the same.
  2. Continued weight shift to the right leg.
D. Head and shoulders
  1. Right cervical rotation continued.
	A. Pelvic girdle movements
	  1. Continued left transverse pelvic girdle rotation.
	B. Rib cage
	  1. Continued left thoracic spine rotation.
	  2. The spinal column is relatively extended.
	C. Base of support
	  1. Slight weight shift to the left leg.
	  2. Left foot is bearing most of the body weight.
	  3. Right ankle is plantar flexed.
	D. Head and shoulders
	  1. Slight cervical extension.

MALE PERFORMER

2. Left shoulder continues through low diagonal adduction.
3. Right shoulder continues through low diagonal adduction.

E. Arms and hands
   1. Left elbow remains extended.

   2. Right elbow is flexed.
   3. Left radio-ulnar joint is pronated.
   4. Right radio-ulnar joint is supinated.

F. Knees and hips
   1. Right knee in extreme extension.
   2. Left knee flexed.

   3. Right hip is at the limit of medial rotation.

   4. Left hip moving toward medial rotation.

FEMALE PERFORMER

2. Left shoulder joint diagonal abduction.
3. Right shoulder joint diagonal adduction.

E. Arms and hands
   1. Left and right elbow extension.
   2. Ulnar flexion both wrists.

F. Knees and hips
   1. Slight flexion of the left knee.
   2. Right knee in relatively the same position.
   3. Continued medial rotation of the left hip joint, but not to the maximum of medial rotation range of motion.
   4. Right hip remains in the same position.

Once the contour drawings have been segmentally analyzed as above, the analysis film should be reviewed frame-by-frame and in slow motion to observe other details which may have been missed between the frames selected for contour drawings. This, in effect, is a double check for the analysis procedure. With the exception of the aggregate muscular analysis, all pertinent and objective information has been collected for proceeding with phases five and six of the skill analysis.

▶ 4. Aggregate Muscular Analysis

In phase three important joint actions involved in softball-hitting were determined as objectively as possible by observing film and contour drawings made from the film. The student in the basic kinesiology course should proceed with a detailed analysis of aggregate muscle actions at this point. These muscle actions can be determined for each joint movement observed in phase three by applying the knowledge of spatial relationships of muscles to joints. As a guide, the student can refer to Part Two or Appendix B. However, it is advised that the student who is doing his first few skill analyses refrain from overuse of Part

Two or Appendix B. There is a need for considerable thought and reflection regarding the myologic implications of the motions observed. The beginning student needs to develop a functional application of myologic subject matter. Once the spatial relationship concept has been mastered by the professional physical educator, there would be relatively little need to do a detailed, written aggregate muscular analysis. The experienced and practicing physical educator who has gained this kinesiologic knowledge through extensive study *and* application does not need to go through phase four in detail. This myologic subject matter has become a "working tool" which the physical educator has incorporated into his professional vocabulary. To gain this functional knowledge of myology, the student must do many complete kinesiologic analyses, particularly of those skills with which he is unfamiliar.

A detailed aggregate muscle analysis of all body segments for both performers in the model is not presented herein. For example purposes, only the *pelvic girdle* and *rib cage segments* are analyzed for their aggregate muscle actions through the preparatory movement and follow-through sequences for the male performer.

PREPARATORY SEQUENCE AGGREGATE MUSCLE ACTION (PELVIC GIRDLE AND RIB CAGE)—Right transverse pelvic rotation is seen. This movement is essential to place the muscles most involved on stretch for the ultimate spinal rotation. The muscles most involved for right transverse pelvic rotation are the right gluteus maximus, left tensor fasciae latae, left gluteus minimus, and anterior fibers of the left gluteus medius. Contralateral muscles for right transverse pelvic rotation are the left gluteus maximus, right tensor fasciae latae, right gluteus minimus, and anterior fibers of the right gluteus medius.

As the pelvic girdle is moved in right transverse rotation, concentric contraction is occurring within the right external oblique and left internal oblique muscles. Concurrently, eccentric contraction is occurring within the left external oblique and right internal oblique muscles. This series of muscle contractions rotates the pelvic girdle to the right side at the same time the rib cage is being rotated to the left side of the athlete as a result of lumbar spine action. Thus, the right external oblique and left internal oblique muscles have been contracted concentrically as a unit, and the left external oblique and right internal oblique muscles have been lengthened and placed on stretch. During these opposite rotations of the pelvic girdle and rib cage, motion has taken place concurrent with relative stability between these two body segments. This is an example of dynamic stabilization—the Lomac Paradox. Furthermore, this is the start of the serape effect. The muscles most involved for left lumbar and thoracic rotation are the right external oblique and left internal oblique muscles. The contralateral muscles are the left external oblique and right internal oblique muscles. The erector spinae muscles guide this action by preventing trunk or lumbar flexion.

MOVEMENT SEQUENCE MUSCULAR ANALYSIS (PELVIC GIRDLE AND RIB CAGE)—When the left external oblique and right internal oblique muscles have been placed on maximum stretch due to right transverse pelvic rotation and left lumbar and thoracic rotation, the movement phase is initiated. The primary movement during this phase is right rotation of the thoracic spine or rib cage and a continuation of right transverse pelvic rotation. The muscles most involved for thoracic and lumbar spinal rotation to the right are the left external oblique and right internal oblique muscles. The contralateral muscles for this movement are the right external oblique and left internal oblique muscles. The erector spinae muscles continue to serve a guiding function by maintaining the spine in an erect position.

RECOVERY SEQUENCE MUSCULAR ANALYSIS (PELVIC GIRDLE AND RIB CAGE)—There is a continuation of right transverse pelvic rotation con-current with thoracic and lumbar spinal rotation to the right. At the conclusion of the follow-through sequence, the left external oblique and right internal oblique muscles have concentrically contracted to their shortest length. Conversely, the muscles contralateral to these muscles have been placed on stretch. This greatly expedites the recovery phase because the athlete must move from this position toward first base. The right external oblique and left internal oblique muscles contract to initiate right transverse pelvic rotation. This facilitates the movement of the lower limbs in starting the run toward first base. This is one myologic advantage of the left-handed hitter over the right-handed hitter.

A myologic analysis of each body joint or segment should be done in this same manner when doing a kinesiologic skill analysis. The pre-ceding example of aggregate muscular analysis of the pelvic girdle and rib cage was done in paragraph form. However, the beginning kinesi-ology student may choose to do a muscular analysis in an outline form. Each action should include the muscles most involved—contralateral muscles, guiding muscles, and the related dynamic stabilizers. The effect of external forces on muscular contraction should also be evaluated.

▶ **5. Synthesis of Anatomic and Kinesiologic Constructs**

During this phase of the skill analysis the physical educator must reflect on all information regarding the athlete. Up to this point, the primary emphasis in the analysis has been on joint movements and the myologic aspects of those movements using as a guide the chart illustrated in Figure 12.1. The next step is to refer to the chart shown in Figure 12.2

"Kinesiologic Considerations for Analyses." These are "recall phrases" from the kinesiologic constructs discussed in Chapter 10. It is recognized that some elements of the kinesiologic constructs will be applicable to some skills and not to others. The physical educator must choose those elements of the constructs most appropriate to the skill being analyzed. Obviously, it is unnecessary to include all three kinesiologic constructs. For example, the softball hitters will be compared and contrasted only in terms of the kinesiologic construct of summation of internal forces. However, a more thorough analysis of hitting might well include both the summation of internal forces and elements of the aerodynamics construct.

PREPARATORY PHASE—This phase is seen in Figure 12.6 and Figure 12.9 for the male and female respectively. The muscle length-force ratio has been more effectively applied by the male performer. His muscles most involved for subsequent spinal rotation have been placed on stretch. This means that the force exerted by those muscles will be greater, because the force exerted by the muscle group placed on stretch is directly proportional to the length of those muscles. The male performer's base of support equilibrium is adequate between the stance and preparatory phases. On the other hand, the female performer's base of support stability is good in the stance, but it deteriorates considerably as she moves into the preparatory phase. The placement of her left foot is away from the line of flight of the ball. Conversely, the male performer's movement of his right foot is into the line of flight of the ball. Movement of the female's foot in this direction causes some slight equilibrium problems resulting in compensatory and extra motion to her left.

MOVEMENT PHASE—Figure 12.5 is the movement phase for the male performer, and Figures 12.10 and 12.11 are the movement phase for the female performer. The female performer's slight lateral rotation at the left hip joint and the placement of the left foot during the stride has resulted in a compensatory movement in the upper limbs. Thus, there is an interruption in the summation of internal forces. This causes a reduction in the amount of force transferred from body part to body part. There is also loss of leverage advantage within the bones acted upon by the muscles most involved. Her arms are held relatively close to the body to maintain equilibrium. This has reduced her muscle length-force ratio within the arm musculature. As can be seen in Figure 12.5, the male performer does not have this same problem. It is also obvious that the rib cage of the female performer has not rotated to a sufficient degree to her right to place the abdominal muscles on their greatest stretch in order to initiate the serape effect. This also reduces the amount of internal force summated and transferred to the next body segments within the kinetic chain.

The male performer is applying his force in the direction of the intended motion. The female performer, however, is moving her body mass away from the direction of intended motion, thus tending to dissipate a percentage of the summated internal forces. The extraneous arm actions noted between Figures 12.8 through 12.10, commonly known as a "hitch," have also caused an interruption within the kinetic chain, resulting in a dissipation of summated internal forces. These factors, combined with the lack of leverage at the point of impact, reduce the bat velocity for the female performer. It can be noted that the male performer has little, if any, wasted motion between frames 12.6 and 12.5. His kinetic chain has been continuous and uninterrupted. Thus his bat velocity at the point of impact has reached its maximum peak. His leverage advantage at the point of impact can be seen by the effective use of his extended elbows. Both performers have maintained an adequate grip at the point of impact. It should be noted that the position of the female's elbow and shoulder joints has a detrimental effect upon the transfer of internal forces through the wrists and the grip action into the sport implement at this point (Figure 12.11). Her leverage advantage is not the same as seen for the male performer in Figure 12.5.

FOLLOW-THROUGH—This phase is seen in Figures 12.4 and 12.12 for the male and female performers respectively. The extent of the follow-through is in direct proportion to the intensity of the summation of internal forces. It can be seen that the male performer has summated a greater degree of internal forces for his swing than the female performer. The female performer has a habit of dropping the bat within a fraction of a second after the recovery phase shown in Figure 12.12. Also, the follow-through for the female performer indicates that she has not used all potential internal force. The left knee has remained slightly flexed, and her pelvic girdle has not been brought over the base of support. On the other hand, the male performer's right knee is fully extended and his pelvic girdle is moving over his base of support in the follow-through sequence.

MAJOR FAULTS OF THE FEMALE PERFORMER—Several fundamental faults have been observed in the female performer's hitting skill. These faults should be recorded in their order of priority for correction, i. e., the most serious fault should be listed first and the other faults listed in the order of importance to the overall skill. The female performer's faults are as follows in rank order:

1. Improper stride—movement of the left foot away from the line of flight of the ball to the performer's left.
2. Limited left transverse pelvic girdle rotation during the movement sequence.

3. Lack of elbow extension during the movement sequence.
4. Lack of shoulder joint extension in the stance.
5. Lack of left knee extension during the final aspects of the movement sequence and during the follow-through and recovery sequences.

The physical educator must use his best professional judgment and extreme care in setting up the priority list for correcting faults of the performer. Experience has indicated that if the major fault is corrected, many of the lesser faults on the priority list will be corrected during the process of eliminating the major skill problem. It is also of importance to deal with the improvement of one fault at a time. Furthermore, all information about the individual, in addition to the kinesiologic analysis, must be used to help improve performance. This type of information is derived over the entire athletic season. Therefore, the coaching suggestions should take into account the analytic findings of the skill as well as the sociopsychologic-physiologic characteristics of the individual. These combined factors would lead to more precise and specific recommendations for the improvement of skill for the performer.

▶ 6. Prescribed Recommendations for Skill Improvement

Shown in Figure 12.3 is a suggested outline for giving prescribed coaching recommendations to improve performance. Particularly for off-seasonal and preseasonal work, the athlete should be provided with one of these charts designed specifically to improve *his* performance. A copy would be kept by the coach along with other information related to the athlete. The following is an example of prescribed coaching recommendations to improve the softball-hitting performance of the female performer shown in Figures 12.8 through 12.12. These recommendations are based upon the kinesiologic analysis and other knowledge of the performer gained over a softball season.

I. "Specifics":
   A. Fifty repetitions of the softball swing with the resistance rope of an Exer-Genie Exerciser attached to the bat handle between the hitter's hands. The initial resistance setting on the Exer-Genie Exerciser should be at two pounds to allow a bat velocity of at least 75 percent of bat velocity used during a game.
II. Skill development drills:
   A. The initial stance should be adjusted to lower the bat about four inches. This can be done by slight extension of both shoulder joints.

B. Stride drill progression:
1. Striding in front of a mirror fifty to seventy-five times daily. Emphasize movement of the left leg into the line of flight of the pitch—left hip abduction.
2. Stride and include left transverse pelvic rotation to the extreme of the range of motion.
3. Stride, left transverse pelvic rotation followed by left and right elbow extension as used in the softball-hitting action.
4. Perform the actual softball swing in front of a mirror, moving the bat through the low diagonal plane of motion—fifty repetitions.
C. Hitting practice.

III. Strength development exercises:
A. Perform strength development exercises for the antigravity musculature (exercises and procedures are discussed in Chapter 13).
B. Combined elbow extension and ulnar flexion exercises performed on an Exer-Genie Exerciser or with a dumbbell.

IV. Flexibility exercises:
A. Spinal rotation exercises, standing or sitting, to both sides through the maximum range of motion. (See Chapter 13.)

V. Muscular endurance exercises:
A. Increase the number of repetitions for the above activities to increase the local muscular endurance of the MMI.

VI. Cardiovascular endurance activities:
(See Chapter 13.)

The analytic process is an on-going procedure performed by the coach throughout the athletic season or year. It can be seen that a thorough analysis of each athlete on film has the potential to allow the coach to make better use of his time during the actual teaching-coaching situation. In practice, the physical educator must rely primarily on using noncinematographic techniques day in and day out.

The complete skill analysis as outlined in this chapter will be of particular benefit to the returning student-athlete who has had the benefit of such an analysis and subsequent coaching suggestions. Each man or woman returning can improve skills during the off-season and preseason of the year. (McKinney, Logan, and Birmingham, 1968) Hence, it can be seen that the professional physical educator who uses kinesiologic knowledge as a "tool" can improve the performer's skill and improve the quality of the performer's motor education by helping him to acquire efficient and effective patterns of action.

SELECTED REFERENCES

1. AKGUN, NECATI, and USTAN, EMIN F. "Teleroentgenologic Investigations of Champion Turkish Wrestlers." *Research Quarterly* 31:547-552, December, 1960.
2. ALDERMAN, RICHARD B. "A Comparative Study of the Effectiveness of Two Grips for Teaching Beginning Golf." *Research Quarterly* 38:3-9, March, 1967.
3. ALEXANDER, JOHN F., and OTHERS. "Effect of Strength Development on Speed of Shooting of Ice Hockey Players." *Research Quarterly* 35:101-106, May, 1964.
4. ARENSEN, ARNE U. "Analyzing the Pole Vault." *Athletic Journal* 39:28, 1959.
5. BLIEVERNICHT, JEAN GELNER. "Accuracy in the Tennis Forehand Drive: Cinematographic Analysis." *Research Quarterly* 39:776-778, October, 1968.
6. BREEN, JAMES L. "What Makes a Good Hitter." *Journal of Health, Physical Education and Recreation* 38:36-39, April, 1961.
7. COLLINS, M. R. "Research on Sprint Running." *Athletic Journal* 32:30, 1952.
8. COUNSILMAN, J. E. "Forces in Swimming Two Types of Crawl Strokes." *Research Quarterly* 26:127, May, 1955.
9. DELLA, D. G. "Individual Differences in Foot Leverage in Relation to Jumping Performance." *Research Quarterly* 21:11, March, 1950.
10. EDWARDS, DONALD K. "Effects of Stride and Position on the Pitching Rubber on Control in Baseball Pitching." *Research Quarterly* 34:9-14, March, 1963.
11. ELBELL, E. R. "Measuring Speed and Force of Charge of Football Players." *Research Quarterly* 23:295, October, 1952.
12. ELFTMAN, HERBERT. "The Basic Pattern of Human Locomotion." *Annals of the New York Academy of Science* 51:1207-1212, 1951.
13. GANSLEN, RICHARD V. "High Hurdling Mechanics." *Scholastic Coach* 18:11, February, 1949.
14. ———. "A Form Study of Don Laz." *Scholastic Coach* 20:9, February, 1951.
15. ———. "The Hop, Step and Jump." *Athletic Journal* 35:12, 14, 16, 67-70, April, 1955.
16. ———. "Style in the Hop, Step and Jump." *Athletic Journal* 36:12-14, May, 1956.
17. GANSLEN, RICHARD V., and JARVINEN, MATTI. "Finnish Javelin Throwing." *Scholastic Coach* 19:8, February, 1950.
18. HAY, JAMES G. "Pole Vaulting: A Mechanical Analysis of Factors Influencing Pole-bend." *Research Quarterly* 38:34-40, March, 1967.
19. ———. "An investigation of Take-Off Impulses in Two Styles of High Jumping." *Research Quarterly* 39:983-992, December, 1968.
20. JOHNSON, JOAN. "The Tennis Serve of Advanced Women Players." *Research Quarterly* 28:123, May, 1957.

21. KING, W. H., and IRWIN, L. W. "A Time and Motion Study of Competitive Backstroke Swimming Turns." *Research Quarterly* 28:257, October, 1957.

22. LANOUE, FRED. "Analysis of the Basic Factors in Fancy Diving." *Research Quarterly* 11:102-109, March, 1940.

23. LAPP, V. W. "A Study of Hammer Velocity and the Physical Factors Involved in Hammer Throwing." *Research Quarterly* 6:134, October, 1935.

24. McKINNEY, WAYNE C., LOGAN, GENE A., and BIRMINGHAM, DICK. "Training Baseball Pitchers in the Off-Season." *Athletic Journal* XLVII:58, 84-86, January, 1968.

25. MAGLISCHO, CHERYL W., and MAGLISCHO, ERNEST. "Comparison of Three Racing Starts Used in Competitive Swimming." *Research Quarterly* 39:604-609, October, 1968.

26. MARSHALL, S. "Factors Affecting Place Kicking in Football." *Research Quarterly* 29:302, October, 1958.

27. MENELY, RONALD, and ROSEMIER, ROBERT A. "Effectiveness of Four Track Starting Positions on Acceleration." *Research Quarterly* 39:161-165, March, 1968.

28. MORTIMER, E. M. "Basketball Shooting." *Research Quarterly* 22:234, May, 1951.

29. MOWERSON, G. R., and McADAM, R. E. "A Comparison of Two Methods of Performing the Racing Start in Competitive Swimming." *Swimming World* 5:4, February, 1964.

30. OWENS, JACK A. "Effect of Variations in Hand and Foot Spacing on Movement Time and on Force Charge." *Research Quarterly* 31:66-76, March, 1960.

31. PETERSON, H. D. "A Scientific Approach to Shooting in Basketball." *Athletic Journal* 40:32, October, 1959.

32. PURDY, BONNIE J., and STALLARD, MARY L. "Effect of Two Learning Methods and Two Grips on the Acquisition of Power and Accuracy in the Golf Swing of College Women." *Research Quarterly* 38:480-484, October, 1967.

33. RACE, DONALD E. "Cinematographic and Mechanical Analysis of External Movements Involved in Hitting a Baseball Effectively." *Research Quarterly* 32:394-404, October, 1961.

34. REHLING, C. H. "Analysis of Techniques of the Golf Drive. *Research Quarterly* 26:80, March, 1955.

35. SCHUBLE, SUE. "Comparative Kinesiologic Analyses of Two Softball Hitting Styles." Unpublished Research, Southwest Missouri State College, Springfield, 1969.

36. SEYMOUR, EMERY W. "Comparison of Base Running Methods." *Research Quarterly* 30:321-325, October, 1959.

37. SLATER-HAMMEL, A. T. "Action Current Study of Contraction-Movement Relationships in the Golf Stroke." *Research Quarterly* 19:164, October, 1948.

38. ———. "An Action Current Study of Contraction-Movement Relationships in the Tennis Stroke." *Research Quarterly* 20:424, December, 1949.

39. SMITH, KARL U., and OTHERS. "Analysis of the Temporal Components of Motion in Human Gait." *American Journal of Physical Medicine* 39:142-151, August, 1960.

40. STOCK, MALCOLM. "Influence of Various Track Starting Positions On Speed." *Research Quarterly* 33:607-614, December, 1962.
41. VAN HUSS, W. D., and OTHERS. "Effect of Overload Warm-up on the Velocity and Accuracy of Throwing." *Research Quarterly* 33:472-475, October, 1962.
42. WHITE, R. A. "Effect of Hip Elevation on the Starting Time of the Sprint." *Research Quarterly Supplement* 6:128-133, 1935.
43. ZIMMERMAN, HELEN M. "Characteristic Likeness and Differences Between Skilled and Non-Skilled Performance of Standing Broad Jump." *Research Quarterly* 27:352-362, October, 1956.

improving performance

One of the major objectives of physical education is to develop the highest possible level of neuromuscular skill in individual students. This objective may be obtained by using kinesiologic techniques during the teaching-learning process. This is not to say that the utilization of kinesiologic principles or constructs alone is sufficient to improve performance adequately. In addition, the physical educator must utilize knowledge about the prevention and care of athletic injuries, methods of presenting subject matter in physical education, the psychologic aspects of the individual students performing, and physiologic principles of sport and exercise. This knowledge is gained through a thorough study of human performance in such courses as kinesiology, motor learning, exercise physiology, athletic injuries, sport psychology, and physical education methods. These courses, and others, are found in any respectable undergraduate professional preparation program for physical education majors.

When prescribing a program to improve performance for any group or individual, there should be a thorough kinesiologic understanding of that program. There must be a basic logic underlying any program of this nature. *The teacher-coach must know what he is trying to accomplish and why he is imposing specific demands in order to bring about favorable adaptations which will improve athletic performance.*

Once analytic procedures of kinesiology have been used to determine the specific changes desired to improve the performance of the athlete, a regimen must be designed to improve the important factors of performance: strength, muscular endurance, cardiovascular endurance, and flexibility. *These undergirding elements provide the basic framework on which skill is developed.* An optimum level of strength is absolutely essential to the performance of any sport skill. Consequently, strength should be the factor of primary concern of anyone who is attempting to improve performance. Concurrent development of these basic factors which underlie performance is feasible and often possible in a well-designed regimen. Emphasis should be placed on what the individual requires in relation to the demands of his sport. This requirement is derived by a thorough analysis of the performer executing the skill. In practice, the need for a given level of strength, muscular endurance, cardiovascular endurance, or flexibility is determined by the professional judgment of the physical educator. This judgment is derived from his professional preparation and experiences.

The development of strength, muscular endurance, cardiovascular endurance, and flexibility is based on the application of the S A I D principle: *Specific Adaptation To Imposed Demands.* (Wallis and Logan, 1964) The demands imposed on the human organism to bring about change in any of the aforementioned factors and to subsequently improve performance must supersede or be progressively more intense than previous demands. As a result of this type of overloading of the organism, specific adaptations result in these performance factors. The imposed demand must be applied specifically to bring about the desired results. The term "specifics," as used in this chapter, is an application of the S A I D principle. *Specifics is defined as application of resistance allowing limb velocities not less than 75 percent of maximum velocity through the exact plane of motion, ranges of motion, and at precise joint angles used by the athlete while performing skills in the athletic contest.* (Logan and McKinney, 1969)

▶ Strength Development

Basic exercises in any general strength development program should be designed to impose overload demands on the antigravity musculature. It is important to give special consideration to the development of strength in the antigravity musculature, because these muscles serve vital movement, postural and dynamic stability functions during athletic performances. Well-conditioned antigravity muscles serve as a "foundation" for sport skill development. For anteroposterior antigravity musculature, the following five muscle groups must be progressively overloaded to develop strength: (1) triceps surae, (2) quadriceps femoris, (3) gluteus maximus, (4) erector spinae, and (5) abdominals. The primary lateral antigravity musculature includes (1) hip area—gluteus medius and hip adductors; (2) lumbar spine—rectus abdominis, internal oblique, external oblique, and erector spinae; and (3) cervical spine—sternocleidomastoid and erector spinae.

Strength development exercises for the anteroposterior antigravity musculature are performed against gravity through the anteroposterior plane of motion. Movement through the anteroposterior plane against gravity imposes a demand on the muscles bilaterally. Strength development for the lateral antigravity musculature involves movement against gravity through the lateral plane of motion. This type of exercise develops strength within the muscle groups most involved in unilateral or one-side movement. This means that exercises to develop lateral antigravity musculature must be done bilaterally.

To develop maximum strength within the shortest period of time, a bout of exercise consisting of eight to twelve repetitions with maximum weight should be done daily. Maximum weight is determined by the individual's ability to complete a minimum of eight repetitions through the desired range of motion. If eight repetitions cannot be completed, too much weight is being used. On the other hand, if the individual can perform more than twelve repetitions, weight should be added to enable the performer to work within the eight-to-twelve repetition range. This procedure should be followed for each exercise in a general strength development regimen designed to improve athletic performance. After the initial muscle soreness, which accompanies any new exercise program, is overcome, the athlete will have no adverse physiologic effects from daily strength development exercise. Some people advocate that strength development exercises should be done on alternate days. The basic rationale for alternating days is that it reduces boredom. However, the motivated athlete will benefit more from a daily program during his off-season. The type of daily activity may be alternated, if desired, to prevent boredom.

Proper execution of resistance exercise should be taught to insure that the most beneficial results will accrue. This should be done according to the best kinesiologic principles to avoid injury. One repetition exercise with maximum weight done in an explosive manner should be avoided. It is true that this is the way weights are handled in the sport of weight lifting, but this is done only after the weight lifter has spent years developing his overall strength. *Breathing while doing resistive exercises for strength development purposes should be done as normally as possible.* The breath should not be held during the more difficult part of the exercise, and there should not be a rapid series of inhalations and breath-holding prior to the lifting of the weight. Holding the breath increases the interabdominal and interthoracic pressures, which may lead to injury.

ANTIGRAVITY STRENGTH DEVELOPMENT EXERCISES—Shown in Figure 13.1 is an exercise to develop strength of the triceps surae muscle group.

A board approximately two inches thick is used to increase the range of motion at the ankle joint. The feet should be straight ahead and placed at shoulder width.

Figure 13.2 is an exercise for the development of the quadricep femoris muscle group and the gluteus maximus. A board should be placed beneath the heels to increase stability. The individual is instructed to perform no more than one-half knee flexion. This may be insured by placing a chair immediately behind the individual performing this exercise.

Figure 13.3 shows an exercise to develop strength in the abdominal musculature. This exercise may be done on a flat surface as well as on an incline board. The starting position is with the heels relatively close to the buttocks, as shown. Additional resistance can be added by placing weights behind the head and/or increasing the incline of the board. While doing this form of hook-lying sit-up, flexion of the cervical spine and

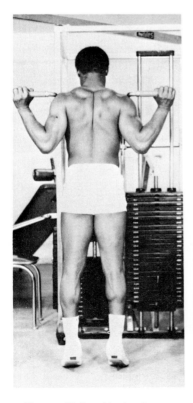 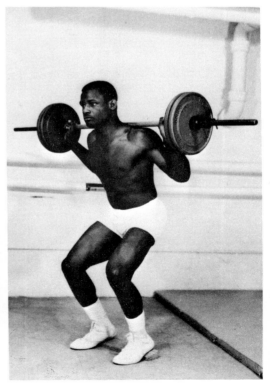

Figure 13.1.   Heel raise.   **Figure 13.2.**   Half squat.

lumbar spine should be stressed at the start of the sit-up. The flexed knees and hips tend to remove the hip flexors from involvement in the exercise. This places more stress on the abdominal muscles, which are the muscles most involved in lumbar flexion. However, when the feet are anchored, the hip flexors become involved in this exercise.

Figure 13.4 is an exercise the purpose of which is to increase strength in the erector spinae muscle group. A padded table should be used, and

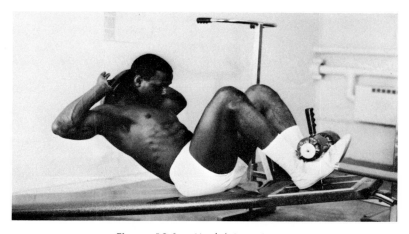

Figure 13.3. Hook-lying sit-up.

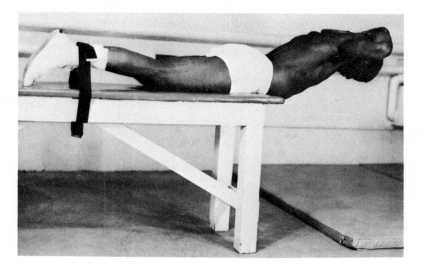

Figure 13.4. Back raise.

the feet must be anchored for stability. A weight may be used to increase the resistance for this exercise. The weight is held immediately behind the individual's neck. During the initial phases of strength development for the erector spinae group, the individual should not raise his trunk higher than the level of the table. However, when strength within the erector spinae musculature has improved appreciably, the individual should go through a complete range of motion.

Illustrated in Figure 13.5 is an exercise to increase strength in the lateral antigravity musculature of the hip, lumbar spine, and cervical spine. Resistance may be added by placing a weight to the side of the individual's head and/or by raising the incline board. Flexing the hips should be avoided in this particular exercise, i. e., the exercise should be done through the lateral plane of motion.

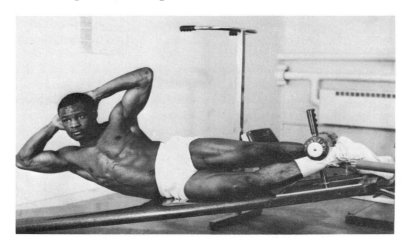

Figure 13.5.   Lateral flexion.

SHOULDER AND ARM STRENGTH DEVELOPMENT EXERCISES—The exercises described in this section are designed to overload the muscle groups in the shoulder and arm area. These exercises are recommended for general strength conditioning. Although the discussion centers around the muscles most involved in bringing about the desired movement at the involved joint, other muscles in the area also benefit from the exercise. These muscles are actively involved either as guiding muscles or as muscles dynamically stabilizing the body areas. Therefore, these five exercises have a beneficial effect upon all shoulder joint, shoulder girdle, arm and related trunk musculature.

Illustration 13.6 shows an exercise which places greatest stress on the latissimus dorsi and lower pectoralis major muscles. The bar may

Figure 13.6. Latissimus pull.

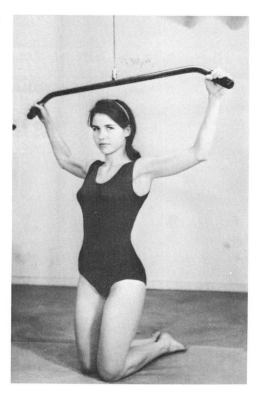

be pulled down behind the head, in front of the head, or in front of the body with the elbows fully extended. Changing the angle of pull in this manner provides movement through different ranges of motion. The body should remain extended during the pulling of the bar.

The bench press is shown in Figure 13.7. This commonly used exercise overloads the triceps brachii, pectoralis major, pectoralis minor, coracobrachialis, short head of the biceps brachii, anterior deltoid, and serratus anterior when performed through the complete range of motion.

Figure 13.8 shows an exercise to develop the strength of the trapezius, serratus anterior, deltoid, and triceps brachii. This exercise can be executed in the standing position; however, it is recommended that it be performed in the seated position as shown. The seated position results in less strain in the lumbar area of the spine.

Figure 13.9 shows an exercise to develop strength in the elbow and wrist flexors. The muscles most involved are the biceps brachii, brachialis, and brachioradialis. Using the pronated position places greater stress

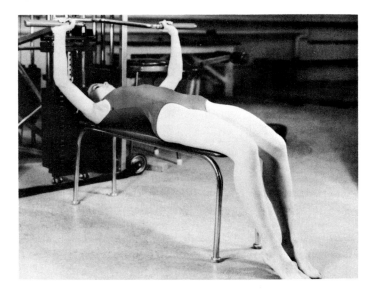

Figure 13.7. Bench press.

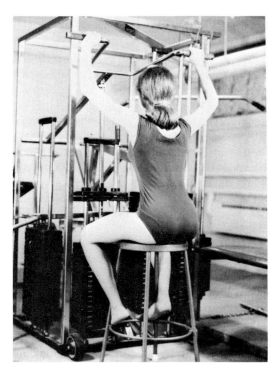

Figure 13.8. Overhead press.

on the wrist extensors. "Sway" of the body should be avoided during this exercise.

Figure 13.10 shows an exercise to develop strength in the triceps brachii, lower pectoralis major, latissimus dorsi, and lower trapezius muscles. The individual's body weight is used as the resistance factor, and this exercise should be repeated for maximum repetitions, i. e., until fatigued.

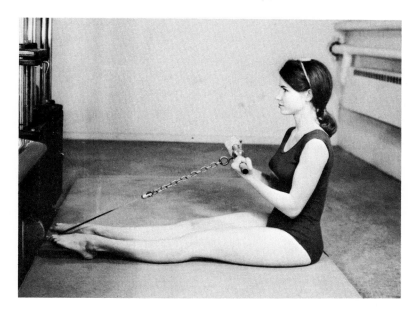

Figure 13.9.   Biceps curl.

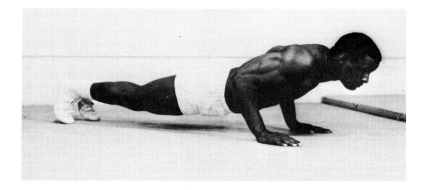

Figure 13.10.   Push-up.

▶ Flexibility

Of the major factors contributing to the development of skill, flexibility is most commonly overlooked in training programs for sports. Flexibility is the range of motion through which body parts move at joints. Joint flexibility can be increased by properly applied exercises, and it is decreased through disuse or inactivity. For normal individuals, flexibility in any joint can be increased appreciably through proper stretching exercises if they are performed continuously over a period of time. Sport performance is inhibited too often by a lack of flexibility.

The SAID principle applies to the development of flexibility. To develop flexibility, the performer must steadily increase the demand on the joint undergoing training in order to increase the joint's range of motion. Contrary to common belief, flexibility is specific to given joints. (Holland, 1968) As an example, an individual's right elbow might be capable of a full range of motion while the left elbow remains relatively inflexible. This condition may be directly related to the work habits of the individual, i. e., flexibility is related to the daily demands placed upon the specific body part. This example indicates that the adaptation of the body part may be positive or negative in response to the demands placed on it. Physical educators have an obligation to impose demands on joints for purposes of improving flexibility and so improve skill.

The optimum degree of flexibility in joints, however, is specific to each activity. Some activities, such as dance and gymnastics, require that performers be highly flexible in many joints. On the other hand, some sport skills require limited ranges of motion.

There are many misconceptions regarding flexibility. The strong, muscular individual may have extreme flexibility in all major joints. Strength and flexibility are independent of each other. Strength involves the state of the contractile tissue within the muscle; whereas, flexibility involves the status of the noncontractile tissue surrounding the muscle fiber as well as in the joint involved. *Therefore, judicious stretching to develop flexibility cannot impede strength development.* Conversely, strength development will not have a detrimental effect on flexibility, providing the individual is working through a full range of motion.

It is recommended that flexibility exercises be done slowly and under control without developing momentum. (Logan and Egstrom, 1961) The use of "bobbing" exercise with momentum prior to an athletic performance may be a predisposing factor to injury of connective tissues during an "all-out" or ballistic athletic performance. It is highly possible that many injuries occur or are "set up" during the stretching phase of the warm-up prior to football games and track meets by stretching the posterior thigh area by "bobbing" with uncontrolled momentum. It has been observed that athletes often limp off the field or track with an injury in the area which has been stretched previously by using this poor technique.

To avoid possible injury during flexibility exercises, "slow stretch to one's limit" is recommended. This slow stretch should be continued beyond the individual's tolerance point for pain. If pain persists throughout a twenty-four-hour period in the body area being stretched, however, the flexibility exercises have been too strenuous. Furthermore, it is advised that the muscles contralateral to the area being stretched should be actively contracted concentrically during the lengthening process. This has a neurologic benefit in dampening the stretch reflex within the musculature being stretched.

There are several body areas requiring special consideration in terms of flexibility. These are the posterior thigh, anterior hip region, lumbar spine area, cervical spine, and the pectoral region of the chest. Connective tissue tends to shorten adaptively in these areas in the inactive individual. The student-athlete is particularly vulnerable because he is generally sedentary during the day. The crucial joint movements to analyze for flexibility are hip joint flexion when the knees are extended, lumbar flexion, cervical flexion, and diagonal abduction at the shoulder joint.

It appears beneficial to precede flexibility exercises with endurance exercises. The rationale for this lies in the assumption that flexibility is more likely to be improved when there is an elevation in the internal temperature of the body. A temperature elevation is a common bodily adaptation which results from endurance exercise.

Each of the flexibility exercises discussed below should be repeated from five to ten times daily to develop flexibility of the joints involved. Bilateral exercises should be repeated on both sides.

Figures 13.11 and 13.12 show one exercise designed to increase flexibility in the posterior hip and lumbar regions. The knee and hip joints should be flexed at the beginning of the exercise. These joints are then extended slowly while the abdominal musculature is contracting concentrically. Figure 13.13 shows an alternate exercise to increase flexibility within the same body areas.

Figure 13.14 shows a flexibility exercise the purpose of which is to increase flexibility within the lumbar spine. The knees are flexed to eliminate the action of the hamstrings on the posterior hip region. The objective is to flex the lumbar spine as much as possible while forcefully contracting the abdominal musculature concentrically.

Figure 13.15 is a flexibility exercise for the thoracic spine. The hands are pressed against the floor as shown, and the abdominals are strongly contracted as the legs are brought back over the head. The knees remain extended throughout the stretch.

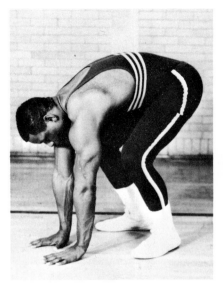 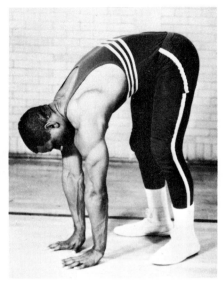

Figure 13.11. Hamstring stretch—standing. Start.

Figure 13.12. Hamstring stretch—standing. Finish.

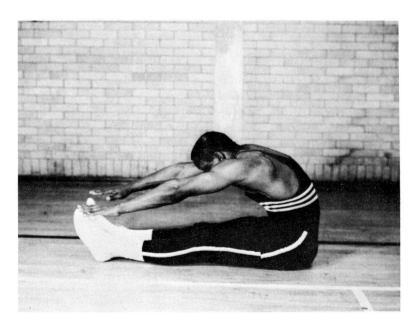

Figure 13.13. Hamstring stretch—sitting.

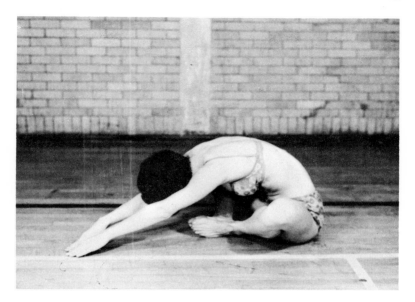

Figure 13.14. Lumbar stretch.

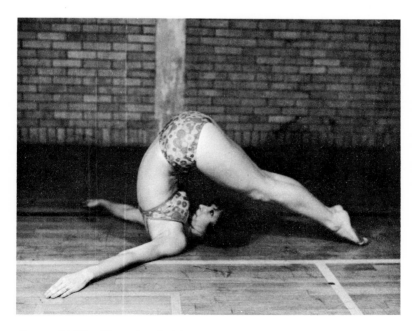

Figure 13.15. Thoracic stretch.

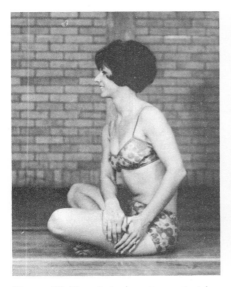 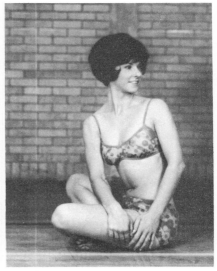

Figure 13.16. Spinal rotary stretch—sitting. Start.

Figure 13.17. Spinal rotary stretch—sitting. Finish.

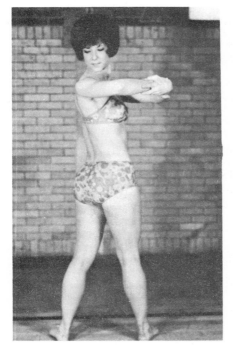

Figure 13.18. Spinal rotary stretch—standing.

Figures 13.16 and 13.17 show an exercise to increase flexibility in the cervical, thoracic, and lumbar spinal areas. Spinal rotation is aided by pressing forcefully against the lateral aspect of the thigh. Another version of this exercise can be done while standing. This is shown in Figure 13.18. The objective in the standing exercise is to attempt to look over one shoulder and see the opposite heel.

The flexibility exercise shown in Figures 13.19 and 13.20 is primarily for the pectoral region. With the elbows and wrists extended the hands

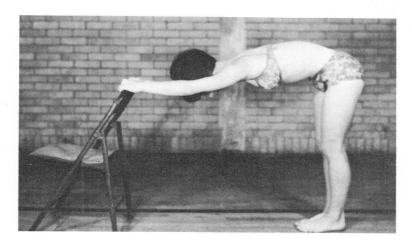

Figure 13.19.   Pectoral stretch. Start.

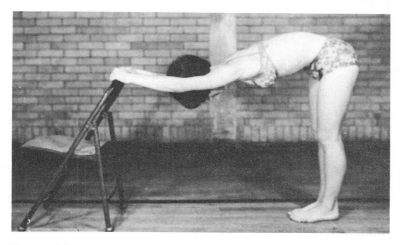

Figure 13.20.   Pectoral stretch. Finish.

are placed on the back of a chair. The head and chest are lowered with a concurrent strong contraction of the abdominal musculature. The knees and hips remain in the same position.

▶ Muscular Endurance

Although strength and muscular endurance are developed concurrently, they are discussed herein as separate entities. The separation of these two factors was done in order to convey ideas more clearly concerning the kinesiologic aspects of strength and muscular endurance development.

A strength-endurance continuum has been hypothesized. (Logan and Foreman, 1961) This hypothesis regarding the existence of a strength-endurance continuum has been supported in the literature. (Yessis, 1963) The development of strength and muscular endurance involves a ratio between the amount of resistance and the number of repetitions. Greater resistance and fewer repetitions will produce strength and some muscular endurance. On the other hand, a greater number of repetitions with low resistance tends to produce muscular endurance and some strength.

An efficient technique for the development of strength and muscular endurance concurrently has been advanced by Morgan and Adamson. (Morgan and Adamson, 1958) Circuit training involves the use of the station method. The circuit can be designed to fulfill the specific objectives of training. Generally, there are six to ten stations in a circuit training program. The following principles should serve as the bases for the development of a circuit: (1) There should be exercises for the antigravity musculature; (2) The stations should be established to work alternate body segments as the athlete moves from one station to the next; and (3) The exercise stations, in addition to the antigravity stations, should be designed to develop muscular endurance for a specific sport.

The example of a circuit training program presented below is designed for athletes involved with throwing skills. There are exercises for the antigravity musculature, shoulder and arm musculature, and a specific throwing exercise through the high diagonal plane of motion against resistance. Resistance loads in a circuit training program are arbitrarily established depending upon the strength and endurance levels of the individuals involved in the group. The strength and muscular endurance levels of the weakest and strongest individuals in the group are taken into consideration when establishing resistance loads. Arbitrarily, the repetition range in a circuit training program should be between ten and thirty repetitions at each station. If the individual with a low level of strength and muscular endurance cannot complete ten repetitions, he should perform his maximum number at the station. On the other hand, if the individual with a high level of strength and muscular endurance can do more than thirty repetitions at a given station, a duplicate station with a higher level of resistance should be provided to allow this person to work between the ten and thirty repetition range.

CIRCUIT TRAINING PROGRAM—The example circuit training program below consists of seven stations: (1) upright rowing, (2) half squat, (3) bench press, (4) flexed knee sit-up, (5) pull-up, (6) back-raise, and (7) throwing.

Station 1, Figure 13.21, shows the upright rowing exercise. The muscles most involved in this exercise are the deltoid, supraspinatus, serratus anterior, biceps brachii, brachialis, brachioradialis, and trapezius.

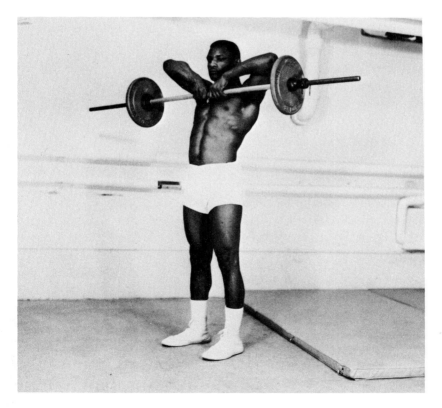

Figure 13.21. Upright rowing—station one.

Station 2, Figure 13.22, is an exercise to develop strength primarily in the quadriceps femoris muscle group. The muscles most involved in the half-squat exercise are the gluteus maximus, rectus femoris, vastus medialis, vastus intermedius, and vastus lateralis muscles. The feet should be shoulder-width apart and the heels are placed on a two-inch board as shown. Also, for safety purposes, a chair is placed behind the athlete to insure half-knee flexion only. Spotters are necessary for this particular exercise to remove the weight from the participant's shoulders if a weight rack is not available.

Station 3, Figure 13.23, shows the bench press. The muscles most involved during the bench press are triceps brachii, pectoralis major, pectoralis minor, coracobrachialis, short head of the biceps brachii, anterior deltoid, and serratus anterior. Spotters are also needed for this particular exercise if weights are used as shown.

Station 4, Figure 13.24, shows the flexed knee sit-up on an incline board. The muscles most involved are the rectus abdominis, external oblique, internal oblique, and transverse abdominis. The resistances for this exercise are applied by changing the angles of the incline board and/or placing additional weight behind the head. Both of these resistances can be increased periodically during the training program. Care

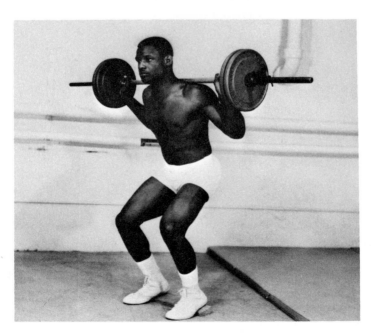

Figure 13.22. Half squat—station two.

should be taken to place the buttocks from six to ten inches from the heels. It should be noted that this exercise is done by flexing the cervical spine and lumbar spine in a "curling fashion."

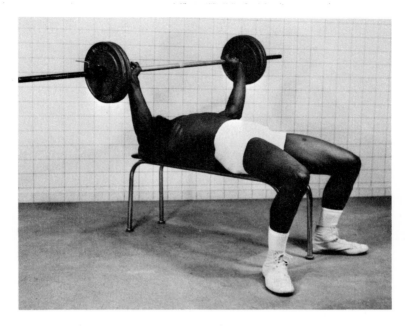

Figure 13.23. Bench press—station three.

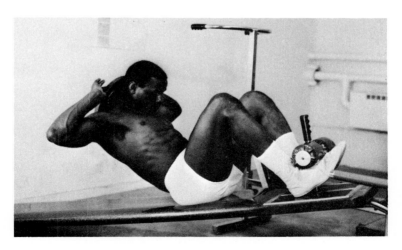

Figure 13.24. Hook-lying sit-up—station four.

Station 5, Figure 13.25, is a pull-up. This exercise can be done with the radio-ulnar joints either pronated or supinated, depending upon the desired outcome. The muscles most involved in the pull-up are the biceps brachii, brachialis, brachioradialis, lower and middle pectoralis major, pectoralis minor, rhomboids, latissimus dorsi, and teres major. The resistance for this exercise is provided by the individual's body weight. If the individual cannot perform ten repetitions of this exercise, he should continue to perform his own maximum each time he reaches this particular station.

Station 6, Figure 13.26, shows the back-raise. The muscles most involved in the back-raise are the erector spinae muscle group, gluteus maximus, biceps femoris, semitendinosus, and semimembranosus. It is recommended that individuals with a relatively low-strength level refrain from lumbar hyperextension. They should move through a range of motion bringing them to the level of the table. Resistance for this exercise is derived from the trunk weight of the individual as well as the weight plate held behind the individual's head. The feet may be held down by

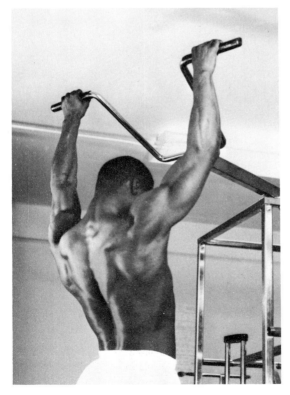

Figure 13.25. Pull-up—station five.

a strap, as shown, or by another individual. Once average strength has been attained in the erector spinae, the back raise should be done through a complete anteroposterior range of motion including lumbar hyperextension.

Station 7, Figure 13.27, shows an exercise designed specifically for throwing. The muscles most involved in this throwing exercise are the

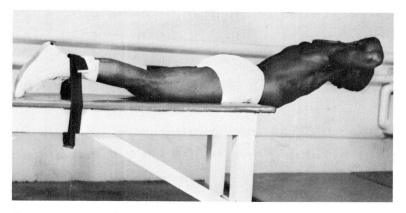

Figure 13.26. Back raise—station six.

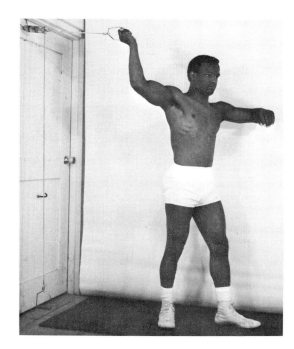

Figure 13.27. Specifics— throwing—station seven.

pectoralis major, teres major, latissimus dorsi, coracobrachialis, short head of the biceps brachii, and triceps brachii. The resistance at this station must be modified on the Exer-Genie Exerciser because this station is primarily concerned with developing strength and local muscular endurance in order to improve throwing skill. It has been determined that limb velocity during a resistance exercise is important to the development of strength, muscular endurance, and throwing skill. *The principle to follow in regard to the amount of resistance is that limb speed during the application of specific resistance should not be reduced more than one-fourth of limb speed without resistance during the actual athletic performance.* (Logan and McKinney, 1967) A greater resistance causes an undesirable change in the athlete's form. Generally, resistances of more than three pounds tend to cause a distinct change in throwing form. It is essential that the athlete concentrate on his throwing form for his particular position. This should include footwork as well as arm and trunk movements.

To start a circuit training program, the squad is divided into equal groups based on the number of stations in the circuit. Since the circuit is designed to work different body segments in sequence, it is not necessary for everyone to start at station one. Therefore, the groups can be distributed evenly throughout the seven stations to initiate the training program. On the first day, all participants complete maximum repetitions at all seven stations on the circuit. These are recorded, and the repetition number is reduced by one-third for each station for each athlete. On subsequent training days, the groups move in sequence through the circuit three times per workout. It is essential to the development of muscular endurance that the groups move through the circuit as rapidly as possible while executing the exercises properly. An example of one individual starting at station one follows: Eighteen repetitions were performed on the first day for upright rowing. This figure is reduced by one-third for subsequent workouts. Consequently, twelve repetitions would be completed each time station one is reached. The same number of repetitions would be repeated three times thus making a total of thirty-six repetitions during the workout period.

The overload demands should be increased as the circuit training program proceeds. This may be done in the following ways: (1) decrease the allotted time for the completion of the three circuits, (2) increase the arbitrarily established resistances at the various stations, or (3) increase the number of repetitions to be performed at each station on the circuit. The maximum repetition self-test should be performed periodically to reestablish the individual's workout repetitions.

▶ Cardiovascular Endurance

The development and maintenance of cardiovascular endurance is one of the major tasks of conditioning. An optimum level of cardiovascular endurance is essential to athletes in virtually all sports. Regular attention to its development and maintenance on a year-round basis is essential. Cardiovascular endurance will regress faster than any of the previously mentioned factors which underlie the development of skill if training is not continuous.

Running is the most effective and efficient technique to develop and maintain cardiovascular endurance. A minimum of fifteen minutes of running three to four times per week is necessary for the average adult to maintain an optimum cardiovascular endurance level. A minimum of twelve minutes of running is necessary to bring about a desirable training effect. The athlete, male or female, must consider twelve minutes of running as a minimum in the developmental process for cardiovascular endurance. This means that there should be a regular training regimen involving running on a year-round, daily basis of periods of time above and beyond those mentioned above.

Any exercise designed to improve cardiovascular endurance should involve the large musculature of the lower limbs. This is essential since the lower limb musculature acts as an auxiliary pump for the heart. It has been estimated that approximately one-third of the circulatory function during activity is performed by the lower limb musculature. This means that running should be a supplementary feature of any weight training or circuit training program.

Running can be incorporated very effectively into a circuit training program. First, prior to starting the actual work on the circuit, the physical educator can have the squad run as far as possible during a predetermined period of time. A predetermined time allows for individual differences, and each individual's distance per workout is recorded. Second, a short run can be introduced following each trip through the circuit. Finally, the training period might be concluded with a second run following the three trips through the circuit.

The Balke Field Test is an excellent and efficient measurement tool for determining the individual's level of cardiovascular fitness. This test consists of running as far as possible within a twelve-minute period of time. (Balke, 1954; Balke and Ware, 1959) Balke's original work has been modified by Kenneth H. Cooper. His modification appears in *Aerobics*. (Cooper, 1968) The norms published by Dr. Cooper are based on the average male adult in a United States Air Force population. Consequently, it is expected that the athlete in excellent cardiovascular condition should exceed the standards established for Cooper's excellent category on the twelve-minute field performance test.

A thorough discussion of cardiovascular endurance is beyond the scope of a basic kinesiology textbook. The reader is referred to exercise physiology textbooks for a more thorough discussion of the development and maintenance of cardiovascular endurance. (Falls, 1968; Karpovich, 1965; Morehouse and Miller, 1967; de Vries, 1966)

▶ Specifics

The traditional weight training exercises utilize movements primarily through the three traditional planes of motion. From an athletic standpoint, this appears to be very unrealistic. For example, some coaches advocate the military press as a beneficial exercise for shot-putters. How many shot-putters put the shot through a transverse plane of motion? A shot is put through a low diagonal plane of motion involving the shoulder joint! Consequently, it is more logical to have the shot-putter use the "Specifics" concept of resistance training. This is not to say that traditional weight training is not potentially beneficial to athletic performance. (Thompson and Martin, 1964) However, "Specifics" are more effective in the actual athletic situation. (Logan and McKinney, 1967; Logan and McKinney, 1969; Logan, McKinney, Rowe, and Lumpe, 1966)

The following steps, for example, would be used prior to placing a shot-putter on a "Specifics" program: (1) analyze his shot-putting style cinematographically to determine major joint angles used during performance; (2) design a weight training program to emphasize strength development of the antigravity musculature, and (3) determine specific resistance exercises through the low diagonal plane of the shoulder, precise joint ranges of motion, and the accurate joint angles utilized during the putting of the shot. Thus, the ideal resistance training program should include general weight training exercises for the antigravity musculature, as well as specific resistance exercises directly related to the skill involved.

All squad members can benefit from the antigravity weight training exercises. There is also a definite need for specific prescribed exercises for each athlete, depending upon the position he plays in his particular sport. The latter concepts require a keen utilization of analytic kinesiology and "Specifics" on the part of the physical educator.

The athlete should work on skill development concurrently with resistance training. It is illogical, especially with athletes involved in accuracy skills, to disregard individual skill development while gaining strength, muscular endurance, cardiovascular endurance, and flexibility. It is recommended that a daily workout program include skill drills as well as resistance training. *This is important because it gives the athlete the opportunity to adjust his skills gradually to anatomic and physiologic changes occurring as a result of his training regimen.* "Specifics" has the distinct advantage of allowing the athlete to concentrate on his form while he is attempting to increase simultaneously strength and flexibility during resistance training. In addition to the development of these factors, the athlete should also concentrate on other skill elements such as footwork.

Specific conditioning can be accomplished by using traditional weight training exercises and equipment, but there are limitations. For example, a traditional pull-over may be modified by using a dumbbell in a motion diagonal to the body. This would appear to be the same type of throwing motion used by a pitcher or outfielder. The main disadvantage is that the athlete is in a back-lying position while doing the pull-over. If he were standing, gravity would do most of the work. The pull-over is unlike throwing in the standing position. The motion, although it resembles throwing, differs completely from a baseball throw. The athlete must use muscle action to stop the momentum of the dumbbell before it strikes his body. This muscular effort is performed at a point far beyond the normal release position of the ball. In addition, the athlete must recover the weight and return it to the starting position or move the weight back through diagonal abduction. Motion against resistance in this case is in direct opposition to the follow-through action of the arm during the throwing process. Also, in the back-lying position no opportunity is present for rotation of the spine or "opening of the hips" (left transverse rotation), which is one of the most important sources of internal force required for throwing with any degree of velocity.

In order to closely duplicate the pitch or throw in this example, the resistance must be carried through the complete range of motion for the throw. This will allow normal striding, medial and lateral rotations at the hip joint, medial rotation of the throwing limb, and movement through the high diagonal plane at the shoulder. There should be no resistance at the conclusion of the follow-through. One isotonic resistance device which allows for the application of "Specifics" is the Exer-Genie Exerciser.[1]

Specific resistance can be used for conditioning athletes in a wide variety of sport skills. It is essential to use cinematographic analysis prior to establishing a program of "Specifics." Cinematographic analysis is more appropriate for the more skilled athlete for purposes of determining "Specifics" than for the lower-level performers. Ideally, the cinema-

---

1. Exer-Genie Exerciser is a registered trademark which identifies this exerciser.

tographic analysis should be made from game film rather than from practice film. As skill increases, there is usually observed a unique or individual style of motion. This individuality of the athlete must be considered when planning training programs for his improvement. From the cinematographic analysis, the physical educator should determine the important planes of motion, ranges of motion, joint angles and body or limb velocity from which to base the subsequent specific training program. This information is used subsequently to attempt to alter performance, especially in the athlete's preseasonal and off-seasonal conditioning programs.

Shown in Figures 13.28 through 13.32 are examples of the application of Specifics. A note of caution is in order in regard to the amount of resistance to be applied during "Specifics" training. A high amount of isotonic resistance is not indicated because of the undesirable changes in form which it will cause. Furthermore, there is also the possibility of muscle and joint damage owing to the fact that joints during ballistic actions are often in positions of mechanical disadvantage. This is also the reason for never applying an "isometric hold" at a point within a

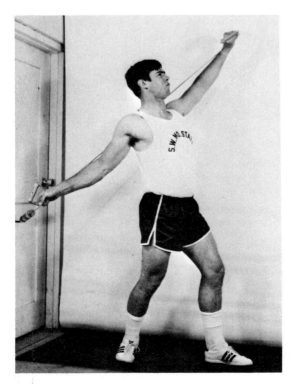

Figure 13.28. Specifics—discus throw through the low diagonal plane.

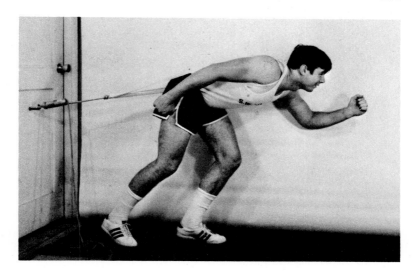

Figure 13.29. Specifics—track start.

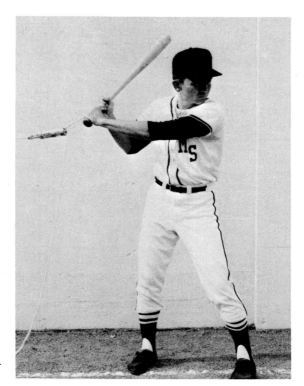

Figure 13.30. Specifics—
baseball hitting.

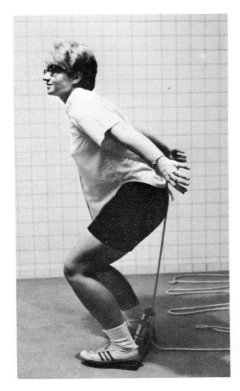

Figure 13.31. Specifics—basketball rebound.

Figure 13.32. Specifics—soccer kick through the diagonal plane at the hip joint.

throwing or kicking range of motion. In addition to the injury potential of the "isometric hold," the movement pattern of the skill is changed. In terms of "Specifics," this is contraindicated for the improvement of skill. *Improvement of skill is one of the major purposes of kinesiology.*

SELECTED REFERENCES

1. BALKE, BRUNO. "Optimal Working Capacity, Its Measurement, and Alteration as Effect of Physical Fatigue." *Arbeitsphysiologie* 15:311, 1954.
2. BALKE, BRUNO, and WARE, RAY W. "The Present Status of Physical Fitness in the Air Force." Air University, Randolph Air Force Base, Texas. School of Aviation Medicine, U.S.A.F., May, 1959.
3. BENDER, JAY A., and KAPLAN, HAROLD M. "The Multiple Angle Testing Method for the Evaluation of Muscle Strength." *Journal of Bone and Joint Surgery* 45A:135-140, January, 1963.

4. BERGER, RICHARD A. "Comparison Between Resistance Load and Strength Improvement." *Research Quarterly* 33:637, December, 1962.
5. BROSE, DONALD E., and HANSON, DALE L. "Effect of Overload Training on Velocity and Accuracy in Throwing." *Research Quarterly* 38:528-533, December, 1967.
6. CLARKE, DAVID H., and HENRY, FRANKLIN M. "Neuromotor Specificity and Increased Speed from Strength Development." *Research Quarterly* 32:315-325, October, 1961.
7. COOPER, KENNETH H. *Aerobics.* New York: M. Evans & Co., Inc., 1968.
8. DAUGHERTY, G. "The Effects of Kinesiological Teaching on the Performance of Junior High School Boys." *Research Quarterly* 16:26, March, 1945.
9. DE VRIES, HERBERT A. "Evaluation of Static Stretching Procedures for Improvement of Flexibility." *Research Quarterly* 33:230-235, May, 1962.
10. ———. *Physiology of Exercise for Physical Education and Athletics.* Dubuque: Wm. C. Brown Company Publishers, 1966.
11. DICKINSON, R. V. "The Specificity of Flexibility." *Research Quarterly* 39:792-793, October, 1968.
12. DOOLITTLE, T. L., and LOGAN, GENE A. "A Device for Measuring Simultaneous Flexion Strength of Both Wrists." *Perceptual and Motor Skills* 21:121-122, August, 1965.
13. EGSTROM, GLEN H., LOGAN, GENE A., and WALLIS, EARL L. "Acquisition of Throwing Skill Involving Projectiles of Varying Weights." *Research Quarterly* 31:420-425, October, 1960.
14. FALLS, HAROLD B., JR. ed. *Exercise Physiology.* New York: Academic Press, Inc., 1968.
15. GARDNER, GERALD W. "Specificity of Strength Changes of the Exercised and Nonexercised Limb Following Isometric Training." *Research Quarterly* 34:98-101, March, 1963.
16. ———. "Effect of Isometric and Isotonic Exercise on Joint Motion." *Archives of Physical Medicine and Rehabilitation* 47:24-30, January, 1966.
17. HENRY, FRANKLIN M., and SMITH, LEON. "Simultaneous vs. Separate Bilateral Muscular Contractions in Relation to Neural Overflow Theory and Neuromotor Specificity." *Research Quarterly* 32:42-46, March, 1961.
18. HOLLAND, GEORGE. "Specificity of Flexibility." *Kinesiology Review—1968.* Washington, D.C.: N.E.A., 1968.
19. HOWELL, MAXWELL L., KIMOTO, RAY, and MORFORD, W. R. "Effect of Isometric and Isotonic Programs Upon Muscular Endurance." *Research Quarterly* 33:536-540, December, 1962.
20. HUPPRICH, F. L., and SIGERSETH, P. O. "The Specificity of Flexibility in Girls." *Research Quarterly* 21:25, March, 1950.
21. KARPOVICH, PETER V. *Physiology of Muscular Activity.* Philadelphia: W.B. Saunders Company, 1965.
22. LEACH, ROBERT E., STRYKER, WILLIAM S., and ZOHN, DAVID A. "A Comparative Study of Isometric and Isotonic Quadriceps Exercise Programs." *Journal of Bone and Joint Surgery* 47A:1421-1426, October, 1965.
23. LEIGHTON, JACK R. "Flexibility Characteristics of Three Specialized Skill Groups of Champion Athletes." *Archives of Physical Medicine and Rehabilitation* 38-580-583, September, 1957.
24. ———. "A Comparison of the Flexibility Characteristics of Weight Training Perfectionists with the Flexibility Characteristics of Four Specialized

Skill Groups of College Athletes." *Journal of the Association for Physical and Mental Rehabilitation* 19:47-51, March-April, 1965.

25. LINDERBURG, FRANKLIN A. "Leg Angle and Muscular Efficiency in the Inverted Leg Press." *Research Quarterly* 35:179-183; May, 1964.

26. LLOYD, B. B. "The Energetics of Running: An Analysis of World Records." *Advancement of Science* 515-530, January, 1966.

27. LOGAN, GENE A. "Comparative Gains in Strength Resulting from Eccentric and Concentric Muscular Contraction." Unpublished Master's Thesis. Urbana: University of Illinois, 1952.

28. ———. "Differential Applications of Resistance and Resulting Strength Measured at Varying Degrees of Knee Extension." Unpublished Ph.D. dissertation. Los Angeles: University of Southern California, 1960.

29. LOGAN, GENE A., and EGSTROM, G. H. "Effects of Slow and Fast Stretching on the Sacro-Femoral Angle." *Journal of the Association for Physical and Mental Rehabilitation* 15:85-86, 89, May-June, 1961.

30. LOGAN, GENE A., and FOREMAN, KENNETH E. "Strength-Endurance Continuum." *The Physical Educator* 18:103, October, 1961.

31. LOGAN, GENE A., and LOCKHART, AILEENE. "Contralateral Transfer of Specificity of Strength Training." *Journal of the American Physical Therapy Association* 42:658-660, October, 1962.

32. LOGAN, GENE A., LOCKHART, AILEENE, and MOTT, JANE A. "Development of Isometric Strength at Different Angles Within the Range of Motion." *Perceptual and Motor Skills* 20:858, June, 1965.

33. LOGAN, GENE A., and McKINNEY, WAYNE C. "Effect of Progressively Increased Resistance Through a Throwing Range of Motion on the Velocity of a Baseball." *Journal of the Association for Physical and Mental Rehabilitation* 21:11-12, 1967.

34. ———. "Cinematographic Analysis of Varying Resistances on Batting Form and Velocity." Unpublished research. Springfield: Southwest Missouri State College, 1969.

35. ———. "Weight Training in Athletics." Unpublished report. Springfield: Southwest Missouri State College, 1969.

36. LOGAN, GENE A., McKINNEY, WAYNE C., ROWE, WM., and LUMPE, JERRY. "Effect of Resistance Through a Throwing Range of Motion on the Velocity of a Baseball." *Perceptual and Motor Skills.* 23:55-58, 1966.

37. LOTTER, WILLARD S. "Specificity or Generality of Speed or Systematically Related Movements." *Research Quarterly* 32:55-62, March, 1961.

38. McKINNEY, WAYNE C. "Transfer of a Learned Neuromuscular Performance to the Ipsilateral and Contralateral Limbs: Dynamic Steadiness and Speed." Unpublished Ph.D. dissertation. Los Angeles: The University of Southern California, 1963.

39. MATHEWS, DONALD K., STACY, RALPH W., and HOOVER, GEORGE N. *Physiology of Muscular Activity and Exercise.* New York: The Ronald Press Company, 1964.

40. MOREHOUSE, LAURENCE E., and MILLER, AUGUSTUS T. *Physiology of Exercise.* St. Louis: The C. V. Mosby Co., 1967.

41. MORGAN, R. E., and ADAMSON, G. T. *Circuit Training.* New Rochelle, New York: Sportshelf and Soccer Associates, 1958.

42. NUNNEY, DEREK N. "Relation of Circuit Training to Swimming." *Research Quarterly* 31:183-198, May, 1960.

43. PIERSON, WILLIAM R., and RASCH, PHILIP J. "Strength and Speed." *Perceptual and Motor Skills* 14:144, February, 1962.
44. SHELTON, ROBERT. Personal Correspondence to Gene A. Logan, 1960.
45. STRAUB, WILLIAM F. "Effect of Overload Training Procedures Upon Velocity and Accuracy of the Overarm Throw." *Research Quarterly* 39:370-379, May, 1968.
46. THOMPSON, C. W., and MARTIN, E. T. "Weight Training and Baseball Throwing Speed." *Journal of the Association for Physical and Mental Rehabilitation* 19:194-196, November-December, 1965.
47. WALLIS, EARL L., and LOGAN, GENE A. *Figure Improvement and Body Conditioning Through Exercise.* Englewood Cliffs: Prentice-Hall, Inc., 1964.
48. WATKINS, DAVID L. "Motion Pictures as an Aid in Correcting Baseball Batting Faults." *Research Quarterly* 34:228-233, May, 1963.
49. WILLIAMS, MARIAN, and STUTZMAN, LEON. "Strength Variation Through the Range of Joint Motion." *Physical Therapy Review* 39:145-152, March, 1959.
50. YESSIS, MICHAEL. "Relationships Between Varying Combinations of Resistances and Repetitions in the Strength-Endurance Continuum." Unpublished Ph.D. dissertation, University of Southern California, 1963.
51. ZAJACZKOWSKA, A. "Constant Velocity in Lifting as a Criterion of Muscular Skill." *Ergonomics* 5:337-356, April, 1962.
52. ZORBAS, W. S., and KARPOVICH, P. V. "The Effect of Weight Lifting Upon the Speed of Muscular Contractions." *Research Quarterly* 22:145, May, 1951.

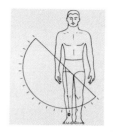

appendixes

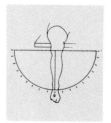

skeletal landmarks and bones

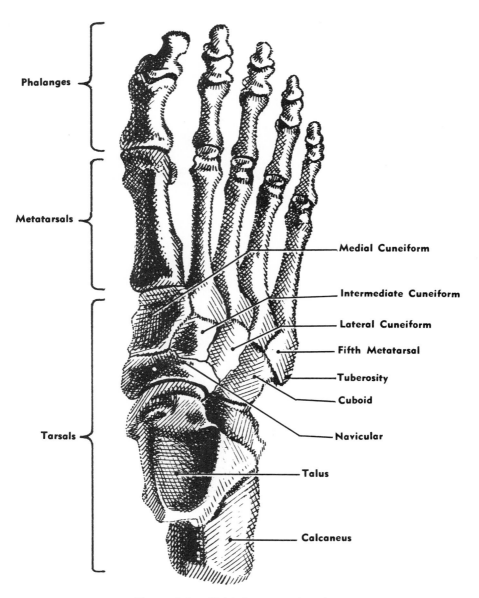

Phalanges

Metatarsals

Tarsals

Medial Cuneiform

Intermediate Cuneiform

Lateral Cuneiform

Fifth Metatarsal

Tuberosity

Cuboid

Navicular

Talus

Calcaneus

Figure A.1. Right foot—superior view.

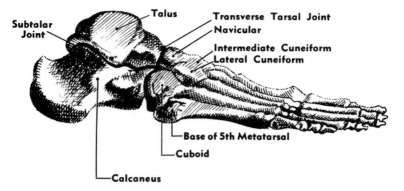

Figure A.2.   Right foot—lateral view.

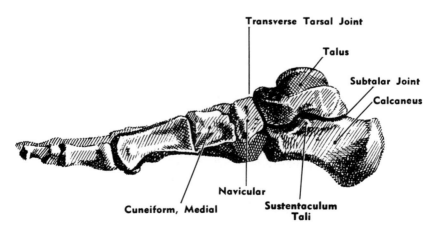

Figure A.3.   Right foot—medial view.

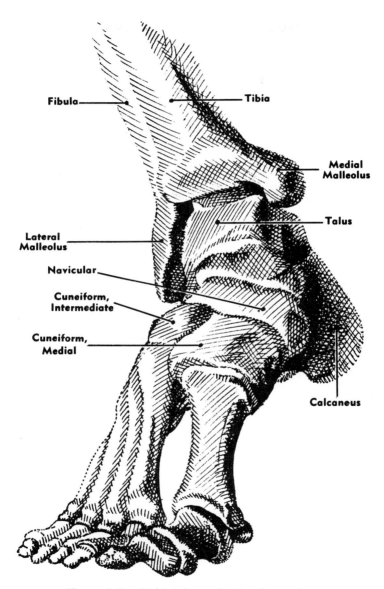

Figure A.4. Right talocrural joint—front view.

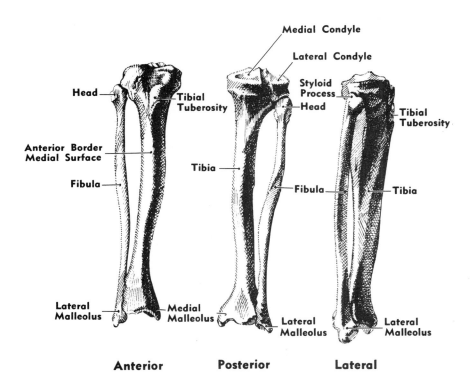

Figure A.5.   Right tibia and fibula.

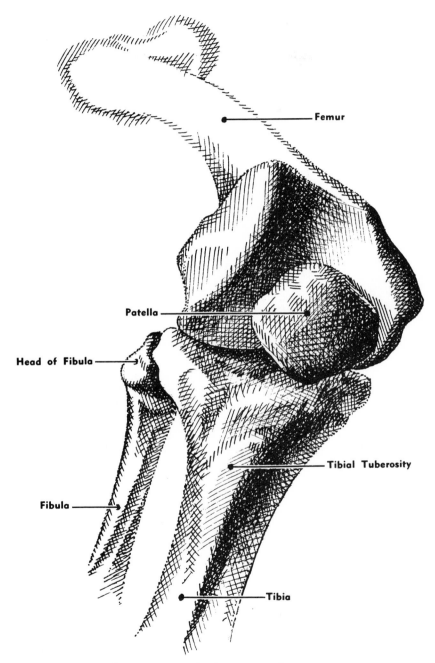

Figure A.6. Right knee joint—front view.

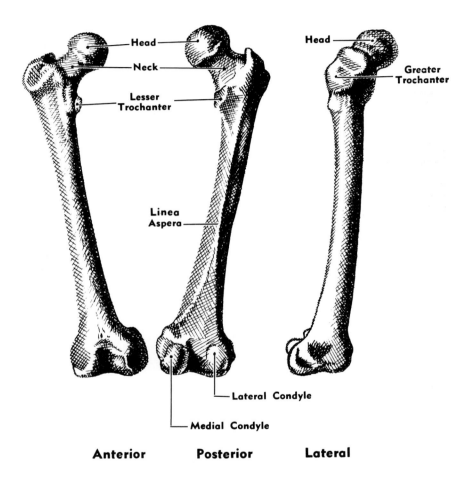

Anterior   **Posterior**   **Lateral**

Figure A.7.   Right femur.

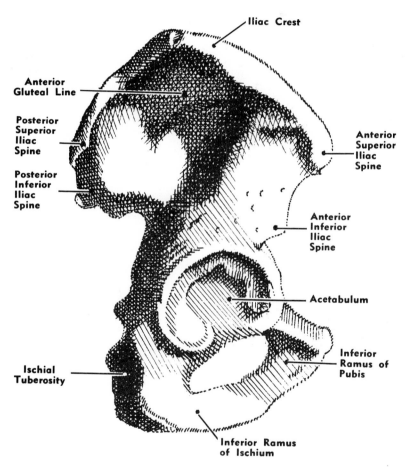

Iliac Crest

Anterior
Gluteal Line

Posterior
Superior
Iliac
Spine

Posterior
Inferior
Iliac
Spine

Anterior
Superior
Iliac
Spine

Anterior
Inferior
Iliac
Spine

Acetabulum

Ischial
Tuberosity

Inferior
Ramus of
Pubis

Inferior Ramus
of Ischium

Figure A.8. Right half pelvic girdle—lateral view.

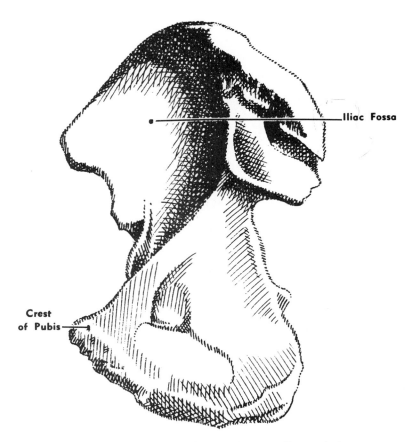

Figure A.9. Right half pelvic girdle—medial view.

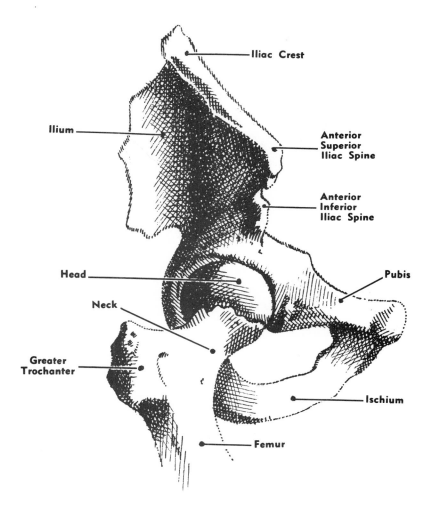

Figure A.10. Right hip joint.

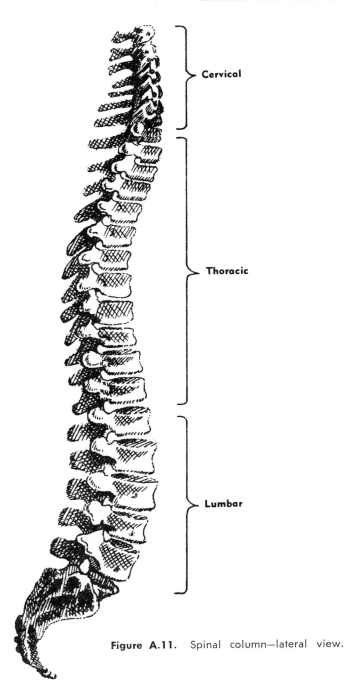

Figure A.11. Spinal column—lateral view.

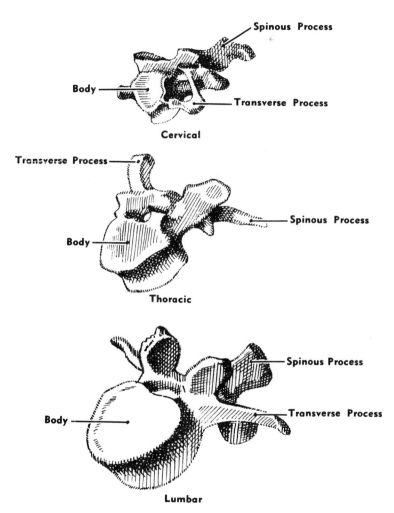

Spinous Process

Body

Transverse Process

Cervical

Transverse Process

Spinous Process

Body

Thoracic

Spinous Process

Transverse Process

Body

Lumbar

Figure A.12. Vertebrae—diagonal view.

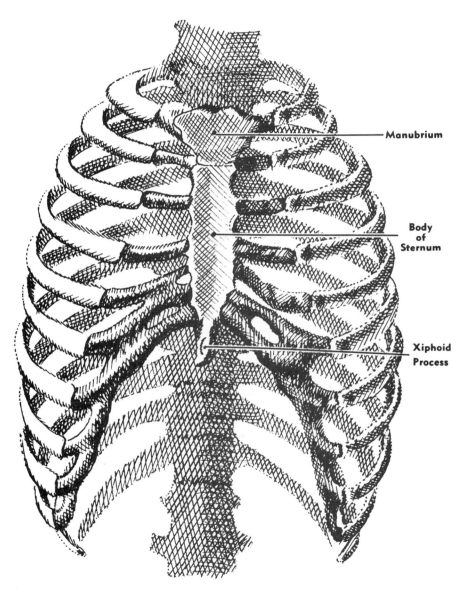

Figure A.13.   Rib cage—anterior view.

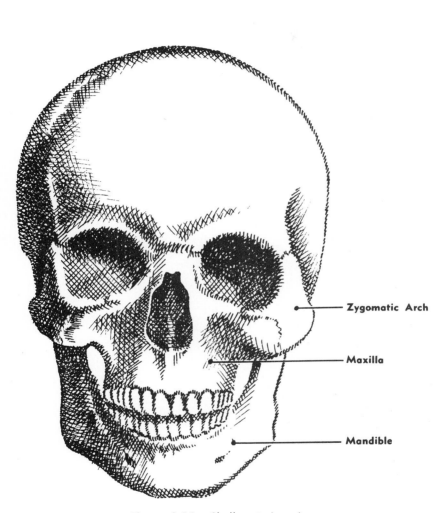

Figure A.14. Skull—anterior view.

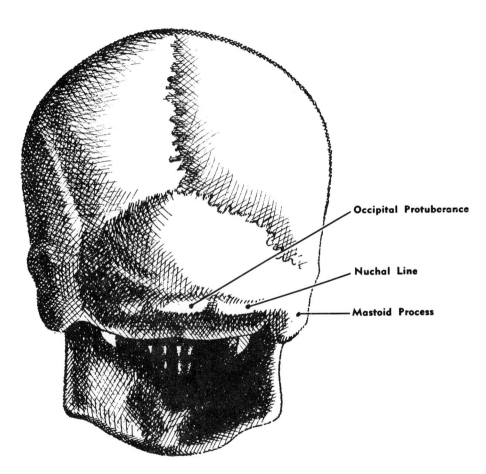

Occipital Protuberance

Nuchal Line

Mastoid Process

Figure A.15.   Skull—posterior view.

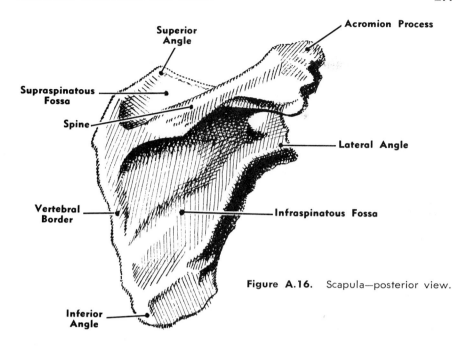

Figure A.16. Scapula—posterior view.

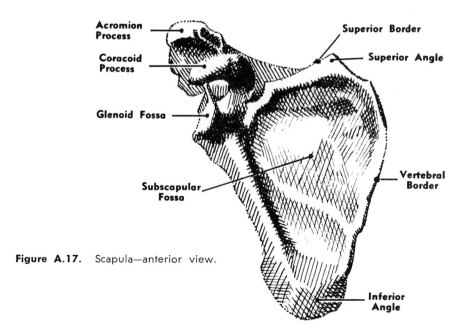

Figure A.17. Scapula—anterior view.

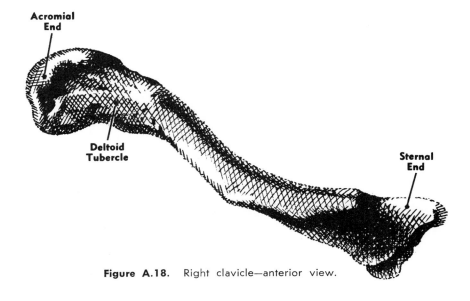

Acromial
End

Deltoid
Tubercle

Sternal
End

Figure A.18. Right clavicle—anterior view.

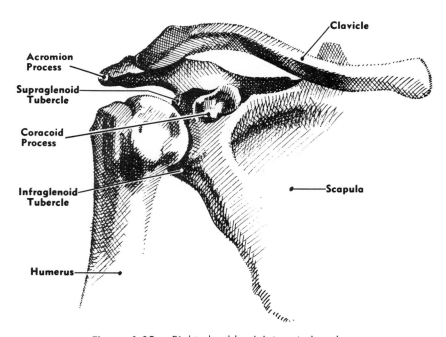

Clavicle

Acromion
Process

Supraglenoid
Tubercle

Coracoid
Process

Infraglenoid
Tubercle

Scapula

Humerus

Figure A.19. Right shoulder joint—anterior view.

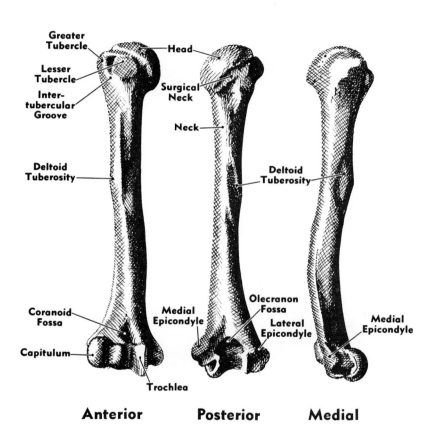

Figure A.20.   Right humerus.

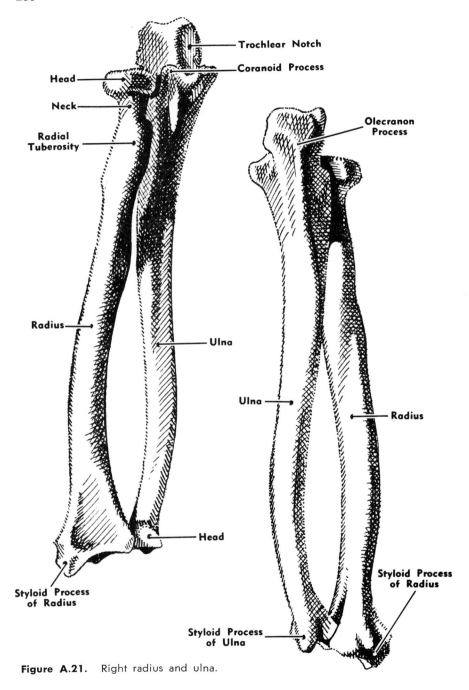

Trochlear Notch

Coranoid Process

Head

Neck

Radial
Tuberosity

Olecranon
Process

Radius

Ulna

Ulna

Radius

Head

Styloid Process
of Radius

Styloid Process
of Radius

Styloid Process
of Ulna

Figure A.21.   Right radius and ulna.

Figure A.22. Right elbow—diagonal view.

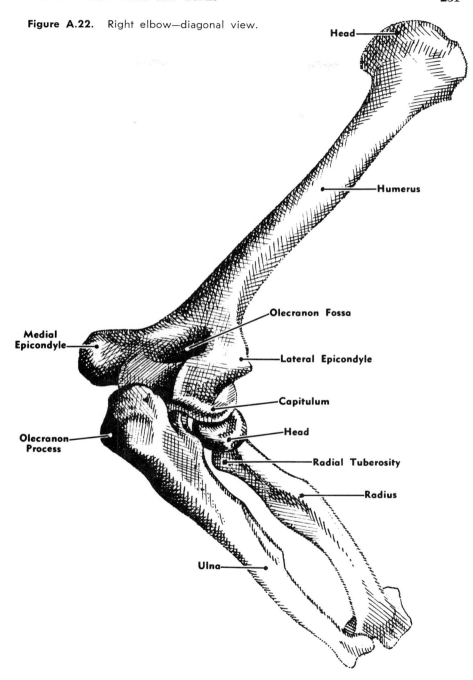

Head

Humerus

Olecranon Fossa

Medial
Epicondyle

Lateral Epicondyle

Capitulum

Head

Olecranon
Process

Radial Tuberosity

Radius

Ulna

muscles most involved in joint movements

MUSCLES[1]	PROXIMAL ATTACHMENT	DISTAL ATTACHMENT
I. *Subtalar and Transverse Tarsal Joint Musculature*—(Articulatio Subtalaris and Articulatio Tarsi Transversa)*		
A. Inverters		
1. Tibialis Anterior	Condylus lateralis of the tibia and upper two-thirds of the lateral aspect of the tibia.	Medial aspect of the os cuneiforme mediale and base of the first metatarsal bone.
2. Tibialis Posterior	Lateral portion of the posterior aspect of the tibia and from the upper two-thirds of the medial aspect of the fibula.	Tuberositas ossis navicularis with fiber connections to the three cuneiformia, cuboideum, and bases of the II, III, and IV metatarsalia.
3. Extensor Hallucis Longus	Middle one-half of the anterior aspect of the fibula.	Phalanx distalis of the great toe (dorsal surface).
4. Flexor Hallucis Longus	Lower two-thirds of the posterior aspect of the fibula.	Phalanx distalis of the great toe (plantar surface).
5. Flexor Digitorum Longus	Posterior surface of the tibia; tendon passes posterior to the malleolus medialis and divides into four tendons.	Phalanx distalis of ossa digitorum pedis II, III, IV, and V (plantar surface).
B. Everters		
1. Extensor Digitorum Longus	Condylus lateralis of the tibia and upper three-fourths of the anterior aspect of fibula and divides into four tendons.	Phalanx media and distalis of the ossa digitorum pedis II, III, IV, and V (dorsal surface).

1. To avoid duplication, the proximal and distal attachments for each muscle will only be presented the first time the muscle appears on the movement list.

*Anatomic nomenclature used in this appendix is consistent with the third edition of *Nomina Anatomica*, 1968 printing.

Muscles	Proximal Attachment	Distal Attachment
2. Peroneus Tertius (fibularis tertius)	Lower one-third of the anterior surface of the fibula.	Basis ossis metatarsalis V (dorsal surface).
3. Peroneus Longus (fibularis longus)	Caput fibulae and upper two-thirds of the lateral aspect of the fibula; tendon runs posterior to the malleolus lateralis.	Basis ossis metatarsalis I and the lateral aspect of the os cuneiforme inermedium (plantar surface).
4. Peroneus Brevis (fibularis brevis)	Lower two-thirds of the lateral surface of the fibula; tendon runs posterior to the malleolus lateralis.	Tuberositas ossis metatarsalis V lateral aspect.

II. *Talocrural Joint Musculature*—(Articulatio talocruralis)

A. Dorsiflexors

  1. Tibialis Anterior

  2. Extensor Hallucis Longus

  3. Extensor Digitorum Longus

  4. Peroneus Tertius (fibularis tertius)

B. Plantar Flexors

Muscles	Proximal Attachment	Distal Attachment
1. Gastrocnemius	Two heads attach to the condylus medialis and condylus lateralis at the posterior aspect of the femur.	Tendo calcaneus (Achillis).
2. Soleus	Caput fibulae and upper one-third of the posterior aspect of the fibula.	Tendo calcaneus (Achillis).

3. Peroneus Longus (fibularis longus)

4. Peroneus Brevis (fibularis brevis)

5. Flexor Digitorum Longus

6. Flexor Hallucis Longus

7. Tibialis Posterior

III. *Knee Joint Musculature*—(Articulatio genus)

A. Extensors

1. Rectus Femoris	Spina iliaca anterior inferior and superior, anterior aspect of the acetabulum.	Tuberositas tibiae via the quadriceps femoris tendon.
2. Vastus Lateralis	Upper portion of the linea intertrochanterica of the femur; anterior and inferior borders of the trochanter major of the femur and upper half of the labius laterale of the linea aspera.	Tuberositas tibiae via the quadriceps femoris tendon.
3. Vastus Medialis	Lower half of the linea intertrochanterica of the femur and the labium mediale of the linea aspera.	Tuberositas tibiae via the quadriceps femoris tendon.
4. Vastus Intermedius	Anterior and lateral aspects of the upper two-thirds of the femur.	Tuberositas tibiae via the quadriceps femoris tendon.

Muscles	Proximal Attachment	Distal Attachment
B. Flexors		
1. Semitendinosus	Tuber ischiadicum of os ischii.	Posterior, medial aspect of the condylus medialis of the tibia.
2. Semi-membranosus	Tuber ischiadicum of os ischii.	Posterior, medial aspect of the condylus medialis of the tibia.
3. Biceps Femoris	*Caput longum*: tuber ischiadicum of os ischii. *Caput breve*: labium laterale of the linea aspera of the femur.	Caput fibulae and condylus lateralis of the tibia.
4. Sartorius	Spina iliaca anterior superior.	Upper portion of the medial aspect of the tibia anterior to the semitendinosus.
5. Gracilis	Upper half of the crista pubica.	Inferior to the condylus medialis of the tibia immediately superior to the semi-tendinosus.
6. Popliteus	Condylus lateralis of the femur.	Posterior surface of the upper and medial one-third of the tibia.
7. Gastrocnemius		
C. Medial Rotators		
1. Semitendinosus		
2. Semi-membranosus		
3. Popliteus		

4. Sartorius

5. Gracilis

D. Lateral Rotator

1. Biceps Femoris

IV. *Hip Joint Musculature*—(Articulatio coxae)

A. Flexors

1. Psoas Major — Each processus transversus of the five vertebrae lumbales and from the bodies of the intervertebral fibrocartilages of the last of the vertebrae thoracicae and all vertebrae lumbales. — Trochanter minor of the femur.

2. Iliacus — Upper two-thirds of the fossa iliaca and labium interum of the crista iliaca. — Lateral to the psoas major on the trochanter minor of the femur.

3. Rectus Femoris

4. Tensor Fasciae Latae — Anterior aspect of the labium externum of the crista iliaca and the spina iliaca anterior superior. — Laterally into the tractus iliotibialis superficial to the trochanter major of the femur. The tractus iliotibialis attaches to the proximal and lateral aspect of the tibia.

5. Pectineus — Between the tubercular pubicum and pecten ossis pubis. — Linea pectinea leading from the trochanter minor to the linea aspera of the femur.

MUSCLES	PROXIMAL ATTACHMENT	DISTAL ATTACHMENT
B. Extensors		
1. Gluteus Maximus	Linea glutea posterior of the ilium and a portion of the posterior aspect of the crista iliaca.	Upper fibers into the posterior fibers of the tractus iliotibialis and lower fibers into the ruberositas glutea on the corpus femoris.
2. Biceps Femoris (caput longum)	*Caput longum*: tuber ischiadicum of os ischii.	Caput fibulae and condylus lateralis of the tibia.
3. Semitendinosus		
4. Semi-membranosus		
C. Abductors		
1. Gluteus medius	From the area of the facies glutea of the ilium between the crista iliaca and linea glutea posterior above and linea glutea anterior below.	Major trochanter of the femur.
2. Gluteus minimus	Beneath the gluteus medius from the area of the facies glutea between the linea glutea anterior and linea glutea inferior of the ilium.	Fossa trochanterica on the anterior aspect of the major trochanter of the femur.
D. Adductors		
1. Adductor brevis	Ramus inferior ossis pubis.	Upper aspect of the linea aspera of the femur.
2. Adductor longus	Cristas pubica.	Linea aspera of the femur between the vastus medialis and adductor magnus.

288

	Origin	Insertion
3. Adductor magnus	Ramus inferior ossis pubis, ramus ossis ischii, and inferior aspect of the tuber ischiadicum.	Linea aspera and tuberculum adductorium of the femur.

4. Gracilis

E. Diagonal Adductors
1. Iliopsoas
2. Rectus femoris
3. Pectineus
4. Adductor magnus
5. Adductor longus
6. Adductor brevis

F. Diagonal Abductors
1. Gluteus maximus
2. Semitendinosus
3. Semi-membranosus

	Origin	Insertion
4. Biceps femoris	Caput longum only.	
5. Piriformis	Anterior aspect of the sacrum and the foramina sacralia pelvina.	Upper aspect of the major trochanter of the femur.
6. Obturatorius internus	Surround the foramen obturatum and attaches to the ramus ossis ischii and ramus inferior ossis pubis.	Medial aspect of the major trochanter of the femur above the fossa trochanterica.

Muscles	Proximal Attachment	Distal Attachment
7. Gemellus superior	Outer aspect of the spina ischiadica.	Medial aspect of the major trochanter of the femur.
8. Gemellus inferior	Upper aspect of the tuber ischiadicum.	Medial aspect of the major trochanter of the femur.
9. Quadratus femoris	External border of the tuber ischiadicum.	Linea intertrochanterica of the femur.
10. Obturatorius externus	Medial aspect of the foramen obturatum, ramus inferior ossis pubis, ramus superior ossis pubis, and the ramus ossis ischii.	Fossa trochanterica of the femur.
11. Gluteus medius		
G. Medial Rotators		
1. Tensor fasciae latae		
2. Gluteus medius—anterior fibers		
3. Gluteus minimus		
H. Lateral Rotators		
1. Gluteus maximus		
2. Gluteus medius—posterior fibers		

290

3. Six lateral rotators

   a. Piriformis

   b. Obturatorius internus

   c. Gemellus superior

   d. Gemellus inferior

   e. Quadratus femoris

   f. Obturatorius externus

V. *Spinal Column and Rib Cage Musculature*—(Columna Vertebralis)

   A. Lumbar and Thoracic Flexors: (vertebrae lumbales and vertebrae thoracicae)

1. Rectus abdominis	Crista pubica.	Anterior on the cartilages of ribs five through seven and on the lateral aspect of the processus xiphodeus.
2. Obliquus externus abdominis	Anterior half of the crista iliaca and the linea alba.	Inferior borders of the lower eight ribs.

Muscles	Proximal Attachment	Distal Attachment
3. Obliquus internus abdominis	Anterior two-thirds of the labium internum of the crista iliaca and lateral half of the inguinal ligament and the lumbodorsal fascia.	Inferior borders of the lower four ribs and the linea alba.
B. Right Diagonal Lumbar Flexors		
1. Left obliquus internus abdominis		
2. Right obliquus externus abdominis		
C. Left Diagonal Lumbar Flexors		
1. Right obliquus internus abdominis		
2. Left obliquus externus abdominis		
D. Right diagonal Lumbar Extensors		
1. Erector spinae		
a. Iliocostalis lumborum	Inferior borders of ribs seven through twelve (posterior).	Crista sacralis intermedia to each processus spinosus of the vertebrae lum-

bales and the lower two vertebrae thoracicae, labium interum of the crista iliaca to the crista sacralis lateralis.

2. Right obliquus internus abdominis
3. Left obliquus externus abdominis

E. Left Diagonal Lumbar Extensors
1. Erector spinae
   a. Iliocostalis lumborum
2. Left obliquus internus abdominis
3. Right obliquus externus abdominis

F. Lumbar and Thoracic Extensors
1. Erector spinae
   a. Iliocostalis lumborum

Muscles	Proximal Attachment	Distal Attachment
b. Iliocostalis thoracis	Superior aspects of ribs one through six (posterior).	Superior aspects of ribs seven through twelve (posterior).
c. Longissimus thoracis	Each processus transversus of the twelve vertebrae thoracicae and the adjacent ribs four through twelve.	Integrated with the iliocostalis lumborum and attaches to each processus transversus of the five vertebrae lumbrales.
d. Spinalis thoracis	Processus spinosus of the upper four to eight vertebrae thoracicae.	Each processus spinosus of vertebrae lumbales four and five as well as each processus spinosus of vertebrae thoracicae eleven and twelve.

G. Right Lateral Flexors of the Lumbar and Thoracic Spine

1. Right obliquus internus abdominis

2. Right obliquus externus abdominis

3. Right rectus abdominis

4. Right erector spinae

H. Left Lateral Flexors of the Lumbar and Thoracic Spine

1. Left obliquus internus abdominis

2. Left obliquus externus abdominis

3. Left rectus abdominis

4. Left erector spinae

I. Right Spinal Rotators of the Lumbar and Thoracic Spine

1. Right obliquus internus abdominis

2. Left obliquus externus abdominis

3. Right erector spinae

Muscles	Proximal Attachment	Distal Attachment
J. Left Spinal Rotators of the Lumbar and Thoracic Spine		
1. Left obliquus internus abdominis		
2. Right obliquus externus abdominis		
3. Left erector spinae		
K. Cervical Flexor		
1. Sternocleido-mastoideus	*Sternal head*: anterior manubrium sterni. *Clavicular head*: medial third of the anterior aspect of the clavicle.	Processus mastoideus and linea nuchae superior.
L. Cervical Extensors		
1. Erector Spinae		
a. Iliocostalis cervicis	Third through sixth ribs posteriorly.	Each tuberculum posterius of each processus transversus of the fourth, fifth, and sixth vertebrae cervicales.
b. Longissimus cervicis	Each processus transversus of vertebrae thoracicae one through five.	Tuberculum posterius of each processus transversus of vertebrae cervicales two through six.

c. Longissimus capitis — Processus mastoideus.

d. Spinalis cervicis — Processus transversus of vertebrae thoracicae one through five and the processus articularis inferior of vertebrae cervicales one through four.

e. Spinalis capitis — Ligamentum nuchae and the processus spinous of the seventh vertebra cervicales. — Processus spinous of the axis vertebra.

M. Right Lateral Flexors of the Cervical Spine — Same as spinalis cervicis. — Same as spinalis cervicis.

1. Right Sterno-cleidomastoideus

2. Right erector spinae

N. Left Lateral Flexors of the Cervical Spine

1. Left Sterno-cleidomastoideus

2. Left erector spinae

O. Right cervical Rotation

1. Right sterno-cleidomastoideus

MUSCLES	PROXIMAL ATTACHMENT	DISTAL ATTACHMENT
2. Left erector spinae		
P. Left Cervical Rotation		
1. Left sterno-cleidomastoideus		
2. Right erector spinae		
VI. *Shoulder Girdle Musculature*		
A. Scapular Abductors		
1. Pectoralis minor	Upper, anterior aspects of ribs three through five.	Medial aspect of the processus cora-coideus of scapula.
2. Serratus anterior	Outer and lateral aspects of ribs one through nine.	The entire vertebral border of the scapula including the angulus superior and angulus inferior.
B. Scapular Adductors		
1. Trapezius (middle fibers)	Protuberatia occipitalis externa and medial third of the linea nuchae superior, ligamentum nuchae and each processus spinosus of all vertebrae thoracicae and the seventh vertebra cervicales.	Posterior border of the lateral third of the clavicle, acromion and spina scapu-lae.

2. Rhomboidei

a. Rhomboideus major — Each processus spinosus of the second through the fifth vertebrae thoracicae. Angulus inferior of the scapula along the vertebral border to the spina scapulae.

b. Rhomboideus minor — Ligamentum nuchae, processus spinosus of the seventh vertebra cervicales, and processus spinosus of the first vertebra thoracicae. Spina scapulae superior to rhomboideus major on vertebral border of the scapula.

C. Scapular Upward Rotators

1. Trapezius (all parts)

2. Serratus anterior (lower fibers)

D. Scapular Downward Rotators

1. Rhomboidei

2. Pectoralis minor

3. Levator scapulae — Processus transversus of the atlas, processus transversus of the axis. Each tuberculum posterius of the processus transversus of third and fourth vertebrae cervicales. Vertebral border of the scapula between the angulus superior and the spina scapulae.

Muscles	Proximal Attachment	Distal Attachment
E. Scapulae Elevators		
1. Levator scapulae		
2. Trapezius (upper fibers)		
3. Rhomboidei		
F. Scapulae Depressors		
1. Trapezius (lower fibers)		
2. Pectoralis minor		
VII. *Shoulder Joint Musculature*–(Articulatio Humeri)		
A. Shoulder Flexors		
1. Deltoideus (anterior fibers)	Anterior aspect of the lateral one-third of the clavicula, acromion and spina scapulae.	Tuberositas deltoidea.
2. Pectoralis major (upper fibers)	Anterior and medial one-half of the clavicula, anterior aspect of the sternum.	Crista tuberculi majoris.
3. Coracobrachialis	Processus coracoideus.	Medial aspect of the corpus humeri.
4. Biceps brachii (caput breve)	*Caput breve*: Processus coracoideus. *Caput longum*: Tuberculum Supraglenoidale of the scapula.	Tuberositas radii.

300

B. Shoulder Extensors

1. Pectoralis major (lower fibers) — Suleus intertubercularis of the humerus.

2. Latissimus dorsi — Each processus spinosus of vertebrae thoracicae seven through twelve, all vertebrae lumbales and vertebrae sacrales; posterior aspect of the crista iliaca; lateral on the labium externum of the crista iliaca and from the lower four ribs posteriorly.

3. Teres major — Angulus inferior of the scapula. — Crista tuberculum minoris of the humerus.

4. Deltoideus (posterior fibers)

5. Triceps brachii (caput longum) — *Caput longum*: tuberculum infraglenoidale of the scapula. — Olecranon of the ulna.

Caput laterale: posterior aspect of the corpus humeri adjacent to the upper part of the sulcus for the radialis nerve.

Caput mediale: margo medialis of the corpus humeri below the radial nerve sulcus.

C. Shoulder Abductors

1. Deltoideus

MUSCLES	PROXIMAL ATTACHMENT	DISTAL ATTACHMENT
2. Pectoralis major (upper fibers when arem is above horizontal)		
3. Suprispinatus	Fossa supra spirata.	Tuberculum majus of the humerus.
D. Shoulder Adductors		
1. Latissimus dorsi		
2. Teres major		
3. Pectoralis major (lower fibers)		
4. Triceps brachii (caput longum)		
E. Shoulder Medial Rotators		
1. Subscapularis	Medial two-thirds of the fossa sub-scapularis.	Tuberculum minus of the humerus.
2. Teres major		
3. Latissimus dorsi		
4. Pectoralis major		
F. Shoulder Lateral Rotators		

1. Infraspinatus	Upper two-thirds of the fossa infraspinata.
2. Teres minor	Axillary border of the upper two-thirds of the scapula.
	Tuberculum majus of the humerus.
	Tuberculum majus of the humerus and upper, medial aspect of the corpus humeri.

G. Shoulder Horizontal Abductors
  1. Deltoideus (middle and posterior fibers)
  2. Infraspinatus
  3. Teres minor
  4. Triceps brachii (caput longum)

H. Shoulder Horizontal Adductors
  1. Deltoideus (anterior fibers)
  2. Pectoralis major
  3. Coracobrachialis
  4. Biceps brachii (caput breve)

303

Muscles	Proximal Attachment	Distal Attachment
I. Shoulder High Diagonal Abductors		
1. Deltoideus (posterior fibers)		
2. Infraspinatus		
3. Teres minor		
4. Triceps brachii (caput longum)		
J. Shoulder High Diagonal Adduction		
1. Deltoideus (anterior fibers)		
2. Pectoralis major (lower fibers)		
3. Coracobrachialis		
4. Biceps brachii (caput breve)		
K. Shoulder Low Diagonal Abduction		
1. Deltoideus (posterior)		
2. Infraspinatus		

3. Teres minor

4. Triceps brachii
   (caput longum)

L. Shoulder Low
   Diagonal Adduction
   1. Deltoideus
      (anterior fibers)

   2. Pectoralis major
      (upper fibers)

   3. Coracobrachialis

   4. Biceps brachii
      (caput breve)

VIII. *Elbow Joint Musculature*—(Articulatio Cubiti)

A. Elbow Flexors
   1. Biceps brachii

   2. Brachialis   Anterior and lower half of the corpus
                                humeri.

   3. Brachioradialis   Upper two-thirds of the lateral pro-
                                cessus supracondylaris of the humerus.

B. Elbow Extensor
   1. Triceps brachii   Tuberositas ulnae and processus coro-
                                noideus.

                                Lateral aspect of the base of the pro-
                                cessus styloideus on the radius.

Muscles	Proximal Attachment	Distal Attachment
IX. *Radio-Ulnar Joint Musculature*—(Articulatio Radioulnaris)		
A. Pronators		
1. Pronator teres	*Caput humerale*: epicondylus medialis of the humerus. *Caput ulnare*: medial aspect of the processus coronoideus on the ulna.	Middle and lateral aspect of the corpus radii.
2. Pronator Quadratus	Volar surface of the lower aspect of the corpus ulnae.	Above the incisura ulnaris of the radius.
3. Brachioradialis		
B. Supinators		
1. Supinator	Epicondylus lateralis of the humerus and crista supinatoris of the ulna.	Dorsal and lateral aspects of the corpus radii.
2. Biceps brachii		
3. Brachioradialis		
X. *Wrist Joint Musculature*—(Articulatio Radiocarpea)		
A. Wrist Flexors		
1. Flexor carpi radialis	Epicondylus medialis of the humerus.	Bases of metacarpalia I and II.
2. Flexor carpi ulnaris	*Caput humerale*: Epicondylus medialis of the humerus. *Caput ulnare*: Medial aspect of the olecranon and upper two-thirds of the dorsal aspect of the ulna.	Pisiforme, hamatum and metacarpus V.

	Origin	Insertion
3. Palmaris longus	Epicondylus medialis of the humerus.	Transverse carpal ligament and the palmar aponeurosis.
4. Flexor digitorum superficialis	*Caput humeroulnare*: Epicondylus medialis of the humerus. *Caput radiale*: Tuberositas radii.	Via four tendons into each side of phalanx media of the four fingers.
5. Flexor Pollicis longus	On the volar surface of the radius below the tuberositas radii and epicondylus medialis of the humerus.	Base of the phalanx distalis of the thumb.

B. Wrist Extensors

	Origin	Insertion
1. Extensor Carpi Radialis Longus	Lower third of the lateral supracondylar ridge of the humerus.	Radial and dorsal aspects of the basis of metacarpus II.
2. Extensor Carpi Radialis Brevis	Epicondylus lateralis of the humerus.	Radial and dorsal aspects of the basis of metacarpus III.
3. Extensor Carpi Ulnaris	Epicondylus lateralis of the humerus.	Ulnar side of the basis of metacarpus V.
4. Extensor Digitorum	Epicondylus lateralis of the humerus.	Via four tendons to the dorsal surface of the phalanx distalis of each digit.
5. Extensor Indicis	Dorsal aspect of the corpus ulnae.	Via the extensor digitorum tendon to the index finger.
6. Extensor digiti minimi	Common extensor tendon and adjacent muscles.	Via the extensor digitorum tendon to the dorsal aspect of the phalanx proximalis of the little finger.
7. Extensor Pollicis Longus	Middle third of the dorsal aspect of the corpus ulnae.	Base of the phalanx distalis of the thumb.

Muscles	Proximal Attachment	Distal Attachment
C. Radial Flexors		
1. Flexor carpi radialis		
2. Extensor carpi radialis longus		
3. Extensor carpi radialis brevis		
4. Extensor pollicis brevis	Dorsal aspect of the corpus radii and the interosseus membrane.	Base of the phalanx proximalis of the thumb.
5. Abductor pollicis longus	Lateral and dorsal aspect of the corpus ulnaris, interosseus membrane and middle third of the dorsal aspect of the corpus radii.	Radial aspect of the basis of Metacarpus I.
D. Ulnar Flexors		
1. Flexor carpi Ulnaris		
2. Extensor carpi Ulnaris		

XI. *Metacarpophalangeal* (Articulationes metacarpophalangeae) *and Interphalangeal* (Articulationes interphalangeae manus) *Musculature*

Muscles	Proximal Attachment	Distal Attachment
A. Flexors		
1. Flexor digitorum profundus	Volar and medial aspects of the upper three-fourths of the corpus ulnae, pro-	Bases of each finger's phalanx distalis.

cessus coronoideus and upper half of the interosseus membrane.

2. Flexor digitorum superficialis

3. Flexor pollicis longus

B. Extensors

1. Extensor digitorum

2. Extensor indicis

3. Extensor digiti minimi

4. Extensor pollicis longus

5. Extensor pollicis brevis

joint range of motion recording forms

These charts are presented as guides for measurement and recording of ranges of motion of major joints of the body. These are intended for general reference purposes only.

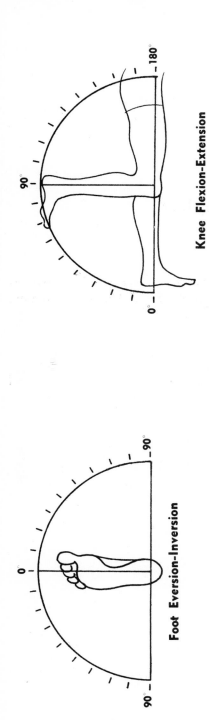

Knee Flexion-Extension

Foot Eversion-Inversion

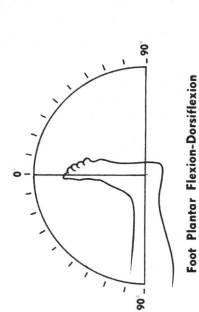

Foot Plantar Flexion-Dorsiflexion

311

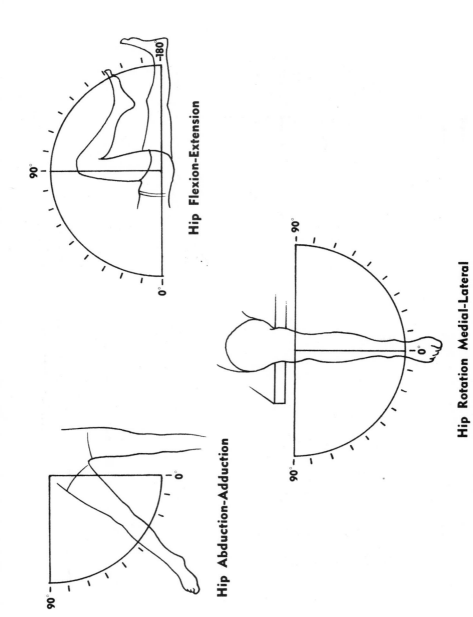

Hip Flexion-Extension

Hip Abduction-Adduction

Hip Rotation Medial-Lateral

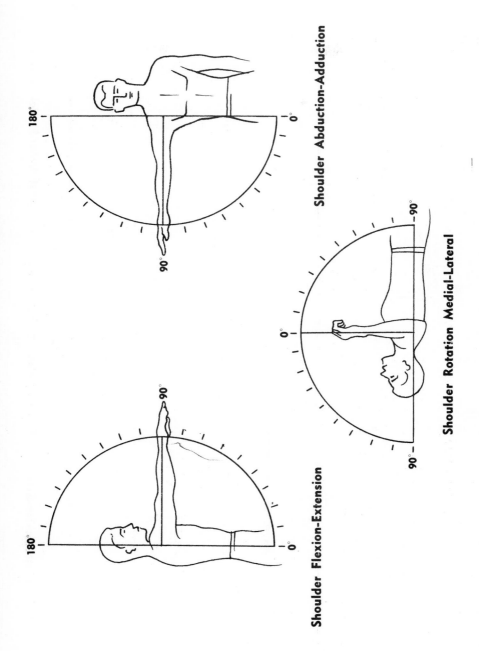

Shoulder Abduction-Adduction

Shoulder Rotation Medial-Lateral

Shoulder Flexion-Extension

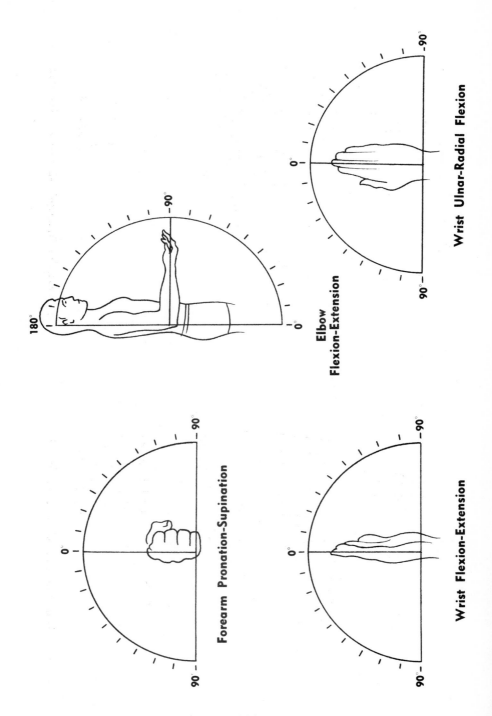

Forearm Pronation-Supination

Elbow
Flexion-Extension

Wrist Flexion-Extension

Wrist Ulnar-Radial Flexion

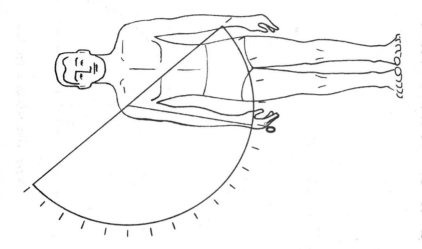

Hip Diagonal Abduction-Adduction

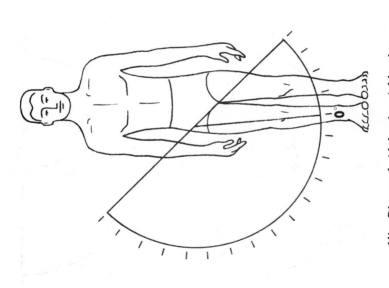

Shoulder Diagonal Abduction-Adduction

index

Specifics, 224, 230, 249, 250, 252-256
Spencer, Richard R., 189
Spinal cord, 60-61
Stabilizing muscles, 59, 71, 75
  Defined, 68
Stacy, Ralph W., 258
Stallard, Mary L., 227
Stecko, George, 103
Steele, Russell W., 204
Steen, Bertil, 103, 117
Steindler, A., 4
Sternoclavicular joint, 33, 118-119, 121
Stetson, R. H., 203
Stevenson, Jan, xi, 256
Stobbs, John, 3
Stock, Malcolm, 228
Straub, William F., 259
Strength development, 225, 229, 230-238
  Repetitions, 231
Stryker, William S., 257
Stutzman, Leon, 259
Sullivan, W. E., 147
Surface anatomy, 59, 73
Sutherland, David H., 104
Sutton, R. M., 189
Swearingen, J. J., 55
Synergistic action, 68
  Helping synergy, 68
  True synergy, 68

T

Tauber, E. S., 204
Taylor, Craig L., 147
Taylor, James, 59, 72
Teaching-coaching defined, 195
Television equipment, 201-202
Thomas, William L., 2
Thompson, Clem, 4, 252, 259
Thompson, J., 104
Tractus iliotibialis, 79, 80, 84, 87, 92, 96
Travill, Anthony, 146, 147
Triceps surae, 78, 150, 151, 230
Tricker, B. J. K., 4
Tricker, R. A. R., 4
Troup, J. D. G., 116

U

Uniarticular muscles, 67
University of Southern California, 15
Ustan, Emin F., 226

V

Van Huss, W. D., 228
Van Linge, B., 147
Velocity, 167
Vertebrae, 105
Vertical plane, 46
Von Treba, Patricia, 204
Voss, Dorothy E., 3, 161

W

Wallis, Earl L., 4, 67, 72, 149, 153, 154, 161, 230, 259
Walsh, Frank P., 103
Walters, C. Etta, 116-117
Ware, Ray W., 251, 256
Watkins, David L., 259
Weathersby, Hal T., 146, 147
Wehrkamp, Robert, 202, 204
Weight shift, 193
Wells, Gordon, 152
Wells, Katharine F., 4
Wheatley, M. D., 104
White, Clarence H., 203
White, R. A., 228
Whiting, H. T. A., 189
Whitley, Jim D., 147, 190
Whitney, R. J., 190
Wilkie, D. R., 188
Wilklow, Leighton B., 103
Williams, Marian, 4, 259
Wilson, Philip D., 3
Winter, F. W., 190
Woods, John B., 104
Wortz, E. C., 153

Y

Yamshon, L. J., 147, 202
Yessis, Michael, 244, 259

Z

Zajaczkowska, A., 259
Zimmerman, Helen M., 228
Zohn, David A., 257
Zorbas, W. S., 259